A WOMB WITH A VIEW

A WOMB WITH A VIEW

America's Growing Public Interest in Pregnancy

Laura Tropp

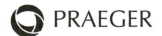 PRAEGER

AN IMPRINT OF ABC-CLIO, LLC
Santa Barbara, California • Denver, Colorado • Oxford, England

Library of Congress Cataloging-in-Publication Data

Tropp, Laura.
  A womb with a view : America's growing public interest in pregnancy / Laura Tropp.
     pages cm
  Includes bibliographical references and index.
  ISBN 978-1-4408-2809-6 (hardcopy : alk. paper) — ISBN 978-1-4408-2810-2 (ebook)   1. Pregnancy—Social aspects—United States.   2. Pregnant women—Public opinion—History.   3. Human body—Social aspects—United States.   I. Title.
  RG556.T76   2013
  362.198200973—dc23   2012033078

ISBN: 978-1-4408-2809-6
EISBN: 978-1-4408-2810-2

17   16   15   14   13   1   2   3   4   5

This book is also available on the World Wide Web as an eBook.
Visit www.abc-clio.com for details.

Praeger
An Imprint of ABC-CLIO, LLC

ABC-CLIO, LLC
130 Cremona Drive, P.O. Box 1911
Santa Barbara, California 93116-1911

This book is printed on acid-free paper ∞

Manufactured in the United States of America

This book is dedicated to Ethan, Maya, and Gillian,
whose "womb time" inspired it.

Contents

Acknowledgments

This book would not have been possible without the advice, assistance, and counsel of many others. I would like to thank my colleagues at Marymount Manhattan College for their support throughout this process. In particular, I thank Katie LeBesco, Peter Naccarato, Anastacia Kurylo, Peter Schaefer, Corey Liberman, Morgan Schwartz, Rebecca Mushtare, M. J. Robinson, Giovanna Chesler, Alister Sanderson, Martha Sledge, Jenny Dixon, and David Linton. Special thanks go to Danielle Berarducci for her eagerness to assist me in any way possible. The college's library staff, in particular Mary Brown and Henry Blanke, were wizards at immediately producing the obscure works I needed. Janet Sternberg inspired this work in a conversation in which she suggested I write a book on the "media ecology" of pregnancy. I also thank those who commented on this book at various stages, including Ben and Betty Hillman, Brian Cogan, Lisa Bocchini, and Kevin and Shulamit Babitz. I am grateful to all the expectant couples and professionals who graciously gave their time to discuss their experiences with me. I especially thank Koren Reyes and Julia Beck, who have both become great resources for me, and Joy Rose and Lynn Kuechle at the Museum of Motherhood. Many people offered ideas or just listened to me talk about the book for many years, including Howard Sneider, Matthew Spain, Melanie Wechsler, Roger and Dee Grabowski, and, especially, Meredith Jose. My students in my Mediating Motherhood courses provided lively discussions, which stimulated my thinking and writing. In particular, I thank Steven Ferezy, who deserves credit for coining the phrase "digital abortion," and Jaimie Sarubbi for keeping me up-to-date on celebrity pregnancies. I also thank the team at Praeger Publishers, especially Debbie Carvalko.

This book truly was a family endeavor. I thank my sister Deborah for helping me develop a strong marketing plan and indulging in my endless conversations about the audience for this book, all while pregnant herself. I have enduring gratitude for my sister Jennifer, who was an invaluable source of advice on subjects ranging from interpreting scientific data to how to balance writing a book while caring for small children. I am grateful to my mother for always offering the-glass-is-half-full optimism and for enthusiastically watching her grandchildren and engaging them in engrossing activities while I wrote. I am in debt to my father who retired just in time to edit and proof this manuscript, and who has spent more time reading the *Chicago Manual of Style* than anyone should. Finally, I would like to thank my husband, Michael Grabowski, who has been a true partner in this endeavor. He spent countless hours editing this book and listened to me talk about pregnancy long after I was pregnant. Truly, the birth of this book would not have happened without him at my side.

Chapter 1

Outing Pregnancy: From Stork to Sonogram

At a cocktail party one night, a friend of ours opened his wallet and showed us a picture of his young daughter. My husband responded in kind by pulling out a photo of our son. This seemingly normal exchange was made odd by the fact that our son was not born yet; I was only six months pregnant. A number of feelings struck me simultaneously. First, I was happy that my husband was so excited and proud about his child-to-be that he wanted to share his experience. I was also grateful that he had a way of becoming involved, other than constantly going to the store to satisfy my varying cravings or listening to me complain about my symptoms. However, I was also a little troubled by what I felt was a small but definite invasion of my privacy. After all, here were my "insides" being displayed to someone else. And to be quite honest, it was the first time during my pregnancy when someone was paying attention to the baby without paying attention to me. I had lost a little bit of control.

Soon after, I began noticing different ways in which pregnancy has become exposed. One need not be pregnant to vicariously experience pregnancy. On the beach, women walk with their pregnant bellies uncovered by bathing suits. When women do cover their bellies, they often use tight clothing that accentuates their growing middle or cute T-shirts with printed phrases that call attention to their baby inside. Far from hiding their bellies, pregnant women now compete in a beauty contest dedicated to them—the winner receives the title of "Missed Period." A modeling agency in Manhattan represents only pregnant women. Sri Lankan rap star M.I.A., nine months pregnant, begins having contractions while performing at the Grammys and no one, herself included, misses a beat. On the cover of popular magazines, celebrities such as Jessica Simpson, Mariah Carey, Angelina Jolie, Katie Holmes, and reality television stars such as "Snooki" (from *Jersey Shore*) and Kim Zolciak (*The Real*

Housewives of Atlanta), showcase their pregnant bodies without controversy, unlike 15 years earlier when Demi Moore posed pregnant and nude for *Vanity Fair.*

Online, pregnancy is everywhere. One week, the most downloaded video on YouTube was a stop-motion animation of a pregnant woman's growing belly, made by her husband. On television, real women give birth on a daily basis in programs on TLC and the Discovery Channel. Once, it was forbidden to utter the word "pregnant" in polite company. Even the groundbreaking *I Love Lucy,* which incorporated its star's real-life pregnancy, never used the word. Now, pregnancy is not only popular, but it is also a selling point. Bravo introduced the reality television program *Pregnant in Heels,* which follows a pregnancy concierge. *Tori & Dean's Inn Love* gained its popularity, in part, from Tori's very public exposing of her pregnancies throughout the show—keeping its momentum, she just gave birth to her fourth child. MTV's *Sixteen and Pregnant* follows real teenagers who find themselves pregnant. Films like *Knocked Up, What to Expect When You're Expecting, Baby Mama,* and *Juno* all flaunt pregnancy as central to their plots. In the television movie *Labor Pains,* Lindsay Lohan pretends to be pregnant and enjoys it; people treat you well, she finds out. Even though the Gloucester teen pregnancy pact was a media fiction, it did not stop Lifetime from creating a film about it or stop bestselling author Barbara Delinsky from writing a fiction book with the same concept (*Not My Daughter*). People enjoy reading and watching pregnancy. Pregnancy is no longer a time to stay out of the limelight but to relish in it.

The celebration of pregnancy has grown to include public acknowledgement of conception. While the sexual revolution of the 1960s opened the door for commercial representations of sex as a recreational activity, conception remained a taboo public topic until recently. A Marriot in South Florida has designed a "grow-the-family" vacation package during the mating season of sea turtles, when couples are encouraged to "fertilize an egg of their own." Instead of "honeymoon" packages, the hotel calls them "babymoon" packages. Elevator conversation in these hotels just got more interesting now that a sexual act once kept hidden becomes the center of a marketing campaign.

This book explores how pregnancy has shifted from private to public experience and the consequences of this shift. In previous historical periods, pregnancy was a sacred time between mother and baby. Only a mother was privy to what her fetus was doing at any moment, and much of that knowledge was imaginary, with the mother trying to visualize her baby and worrying about her own impact on the growth of the fetus. Women were warned to stay away from not only specific foods that might "sour" her baby but also ideas or daydreams that could scar the child. Although superstition governed prenatal care, people at least respected the power of the mother. Long before the power of feminist movements, the mother was recognized as the person with the most important connection to the baby. Now, mothers are just a part of the action. While fathers are sharing in that action more than ever before, the fetus itself has become exposed and available to the public, and numerous products and services are marketed with that in mind.

Prior to the late 20th century, the fetus was sheltered as much as possible from the outside world during pregnancy. Women wore special clothing to hide their bellies, and they segregated themselves from the company of men. In later periods, women further isolated themselves, as doctors and other moral authorities advised them to stay in their homes to wait out their pregnancies. Now, the public's appetite for pregnancy has utterly reversed this attitude; the fetus is constantly on display. Tom Cruise claims he bought his own personal ultrasound machine in part because he was afraid of having his future daughter's image spread throughout the Internet. Women with fewer resources than Cruise can go to a private office and pay for ultrasounds that are not medically necessary. These personalized experiences allow women to see their developing baby on their own time. Often, women describe the experience of getting to know their babies as wonderful and leisurely. For some, it becomes in some ways more significant than birth itself. One woman I spoke with described her disappointment at her baby's birth because she felt like she had already met her during her ultrasound. The experience affected her so much that she chose to forego seeing the advanced medical sonograms during her next pregnancy: "The second time, I opted for mystery," she told me "The first time, it was a little too much information."

Once we see the fetus, we begin to interact with it as if it already is outside the womb. Some parents, anxious to get ahead in preparing their child for the Ivy Leagues, use all manners of technology to "educate" or "entertain" their babies while in the womb. Everything from womb music to a more complicated education system that claims to create smarter babies is available for purchase.

Adding to this anxiety are all the sources of information warning mothers of the risks to their fetus lurking out there. These risks go far beyond the traditional lists of which foods to avoid. A quick Internet search reveals a long inventory of what to avoid while pregnant:[1]

Advice for Pregnant Women:

- Avoid caffeine
- Avoid cats
- Avoid chocolate
- Avoid exposure to pesticides
- Avoid fish
- Avoid junk food
- Avoid lead
- Avoid reptiles
- Avoid stress
- Avoid tick bites
- Avoid VDTs (video display terminals), particularly those that are older
- Do not breathe fumes from paint and household cleaning products
- Do not drink diet soda
- Do not drink herbal tea
- Do not eat deli meats
- Do not eat raw meat
- Do not eat soft cheeses (such as brie, feta, or blue cheese)
- Do not have soft-serve ice-cream
- Do not have vitamin A supplements
- Do not raise your body temperature, particularly not above 102 degrees
- Do not ride theme park rides
- Do not take illegal drugs
- Do not take prescription drugs or over the counter drugs (without specific permission from your doctor)
- Do not use a sauna, hot tub, or take long baths
- Do not drink alcohol
- Do not drink tap water
- Do not eat hot dogs
- Do not get herpes
- Do not have X-rays
- Do not smoke or be around smokers
- Do not stand by your microwave
- Do not use a water bed
- Do not use an electric blanket

Some of these items, like illegal drugs and herpes, seem so obvious for anyone to avoid that one wonders why pregnant women in particular must be warned about them. Other warnings are more controversial, like fish.

Although some studies have indicated that high mercury levels in some fish can hurt fetal development, newer studies demonstrate that removing fish from a pregnant woman's diet prevents the fetus from receiving useful nutrition like omega-3 fatty acids. Other warnings, like avoiding video monitors, have no conclusive evidence to back them up.

What's most alarming is that these lists get copied and pasted without vetting, and women often receive contradictory information about what they should do. I have overheard many a conversation among pregnant women trying to decide whether they could eat a turkey sandwich. One woman wrote that she thought she was already a bad mother because she absentmindedly had a relaxing cup of green tea.

Before I realized I was pregnant with my first child, I had in the preceding month a margarita, an X-ray, and sushi: the holy trinity of "no-no's" for pregnant women. I was an anxious wreck until my OB reassured me that anything that I did that early "didn't count." She said I was "grandfathered" in for those items, as long as I promised to have a strict baby-friendly diet and environment from that point onward. I consider myself lucky that my OB was as relaxed as she was; because new studies emerge almost weekly that offer new and sometimes contradictory advice, a visit to the doctor's office may leave some women more confused than reassured.

In the postindustrial United States, the information age allows unfettered access to an abundance of information, often without a useful filter for contextualizing that data. Women have more information about pregnancy than ever before, but no way to figure out what to pay attention to. One psychiatric professional advises her anxious pregnant patients to get rid of their Wi-Fi accounts because too-quick access to the Internet makes them more nervous than ever before. The womb, naturally created for our bodies to protect and nurture a growing fetus, seems to be insufficient in the brave new world. Now, it is enhanced via prepared lessons and classical music and guarded from any potentially dangerous substance, real or imagined.

The ability to see the fetus has encouraged fathers, family, and friends to participate in the pregnancy process long before the birth of the baby. While this has the wonderful benefit of encouraging early bonding between fathers and their offspring and strengthening family ties, it also seizes power from mothers. Now, women describe how, at the hospital, doctors often trust medical tests and tools over their own symptoms. I remember my own argument with a delivery nurse when I was deep in labor during my second pregnancy: she did not believe I was really having contractions three minutes apart. I felt them (boy did I feel them), but the nurse could not find them on the fetal monitor. My husband was left in the position of trying to decide whether to believe me or the technology (luckily he chose me). Mothers are no longer the primary holders of information about the fetus as technology displaces instinct.

This book is not an advice or a how-to book. It will not tell you what to avoid while pregnant or ways to be a "better" pregnant woman. It is not even exclusively for pregnant women. As this book argues, pregnancy is no longer a unique experience for pregnant women; all types of people are interested in watching pregnant women and interacting with the pregnant experience. With the preponderance of reality shows, surveillance cameras, and a public fascination with voyeurism of all types, pregnancy may be just another thing to gaze at.

And gaze, we do. The blog HisBoysCanSwim.com is an anonymous chronicle of one couple's pregnancy journey. They have 1,000–2,000 hits per day and 13,500 followers on their Twitter feed. When I spoke to this couple, they were baffled by both the number of people who were interested in their story and how many of them were not and have never been pregnant. But the dad found the blog a useful way for him to connect with the pregnancy. Fathers are becoming more involved than before. A male colleague of mine had placed a pink bunny with a pink blanket above his desk. When I asked him about it, he said a friend gave it to him to publicly display so that others would know his wife was expecting a baby. Lacking a belly bump to spark conversation, he displayed the bunny so he could participate in the announcement and share the excitement of others in acknowledging his wife's pregnancy. While his involvement is commendable, conflicts over control of what pregnancy represents are likely to occur as men become more involved in a once exclusively female process. In the past, men would wait to celebrate the birth of the child, but now they also want to celebrate the conception of the child.

Pregnancy may be the latest fad in our culture. Magazines depict celebrities like Angelina Jolie, Salma Hayek, and Jennifer Garner relishing their pregnancies. Tabloid television specials follow the quirky adventures of Nadya Suleman, aka "Octomom," who had such a desire to be pregnant that she went through in vitro fertilization to give birth to the United States' first set of living octuplets, generating controversy since she is a single mom with six other children. Getting pregnant, being pregnant, and watching pregnancy are all in the public mind. However, fads disappear, but pregnant women never will. After all, pregnancy is required for our very existence. This book allows all those interested to take a step back and see how our very notion of pregnancy has evolved.

This book is about changes in how we see and understand pregnancy. The growth of hospitals, the displacement of midwives by doctors, changes in views of sexuality, and the role of women and men in society have all influenced the pregnant experience. The book certainly examines these factors, but it singles out the role that technology and media have played in changing the symbolic significance of pregnancy.

This book is inspired by the work of medium theorists like Marshall McLuhan and Neil Postman, who recognized that the dominant medium of any period influences how a society thinks and acts. For example, the Internet has added a new way of communicating, but also created new social relationships, shifted economic models, and changed our perception of space and time. One friend of mine was having awful acid reflex during her pregnancy, making it difficult for her to eat most foods and rather unpleasant to walk around during the day. Her obstetrician could provide her with little relief, and none of her friends had useful advice. One day, she typed out her symptoms on an Internet search and within seconds had her solution: black licorice. For her, the Internet served as a useful resource; without it, she would have never found relief. However, for other pregnant women, the information explosion leads only to higher levels of anxiety and confusion about how to manage their pregnancy.

Postman argued that all technology presents this sort of Faustian bargain, where culture benefits in some ways but suffers in others. This book is interested in what happens to pregnancy in both good and bad ways as technologies and other societal changes influence the pregnant experience. It examines, for example, how ultrasounds, digital cameras, television, and the Internet all have changed how we view pregnancy. The book also explores what happens when pregnancy becomes more exposed to the world. X-rays, ultrasounds, film, and video cameras have all shifted the ability of doctors, parents, and the public to peer into a woman's body. These technologies can give more power to the fetus, as in the development of a fetal rights movement, sometimes at the expense of the mother's power. It can change social relationships, as fathers can bond to the baby much earlier. But, it also has the potential to commoditize the entire pregnancy process. For example, a pregnant woman recently "sold" her visible belly to advertise a Las Vegas casino. The same company sponsored her birth, providing masks and gowns with logos.[2] Personal baby planners now guide families through the process of becoming a mother. Once something that was taken for granted as a natural process for a woman, assisted by her friends, neighbors, and families, has now become a commercialized experience through the hiring of these experts or the purchase of any number of products marketed to pregnant women. These examples illustrate how shifts in access to technology and the introduction of experts have broad social, political, and economic consequences for society.

This book explores how pregnancy has shifted over time and how it is depicted in popular culture. Chapter two traces the shift from when women could use only their senses and intuition to connect to their pregnancy to the present, when technology mediates that connection. Expectant parents pay for personalized, nonmedical ultrasounds for a leisurely peek at their little one-to-be.

The mother's exclusive relationship to her fetus is lost, but new relationships emerge. Now, there is an increasing desire to move beyond peering in to stimulating and creating a relationship with the fetus prior to birth. Products are marketed that promise to make your baby smarter if you begin to stimulate them in the womb. The chapter details technological efforts to gaze at the fetus and the implications of these efforts for the family and the fetus itself.

Chapter three describes how the manner in which women have received information about their pregnancies has changed. In the past, pregnant women relied on other women for advice about being pregnant. Pregnancy allowed them into a club that was, for the most part, exclusively female and populated by those close in proximity. A number of factors, including industrialization, created a loss of this social capital for women. The book industry produced a market to make up for this loss, and medical professionals displaced women for dispensing advice. The chapter details these shifts and how the Internet is allowing a return to the experience of pregnant women getting advice from and giving it to others. Yet today, the club is open to all and has created a society of pregnancy voyeurs.

Chapter four explores representations of pregnancy in popular culture, where its shift to public space is most apparent. Needless embarrassment has been replaced by pride in pregnancy, and the unmistakable sign of impending childbirth is affectionately called a "bump." Just as the fetus has been outed, so has pregnancy itself. From television to film to the Internet, there is an explosion of pregnant characters in programs and real pregnant women who are filmed for an audience. The chapter details this representation and how it has changed our experience and perception of pregnancy and birth.

Chapter five focuses on the role of fathers in pregnancy. Dads have moved from watching on the sidelines to a more central role during pregnancy. Dads-to-be are now more involved in the fertility process: beyond contributing sperm, they help their female partners keep track of their cycles and search for those perfect days. Once they successfully fertilize an egg, men create blogs to report on the progress of their babies, read literature written specifically for them, and attend classes created for expectant fathers. VH1's reality television program *Dad Camp* shows Dr. Jeff putting potentially irresponsible fathers through a preparedness program, forcing them to participate in activities and workshops designed to test and strengthen their ability to be a fit parent. Other programs follow the life transition of former television stars like Scott Baio and Mario Lopez as they prepare to become fathers. Shows like this showcase expectant fatherhood as a new life stage to be undertaken by dads and capitalized on by marketers.

Chapter six considers the celebrity pregnant experience and the changing world of maternity fashion. Tracing changing representations of pregnancy in *People* magazine, the chapter shows how celebrities have shifted from hiding their pregnancies to exposing them. Demi Moore is remembered for the moment when she bared her belly for all to see, but what historical and technological breakthroughs preceded Moore that allowed her that moment? The chapter also examines how fans follow celebrity pregnancies. When Jennifer Lopez announced she was pregnant at a concert with her husband, Marc Anthony, the moment was captured and posted on YouTube by an adoring fan. Websites allow fans to follow the "baby bump" on their favorite celebrity. The chapter also examines how maternity fashions, often first shown off by celebrities, have changed to a look that encourages women to show off their pregnancy. The chapter looks at new trends in pregnancy fashion. A branding firm now specializes in marketing to pregnant women, and some popular designers are beginning to design maternity lines. In some ways, fashion has taken on the specter of ritual, as pregnant women promote trends like belly molds and belly painting as part of their own personal ceremonies. The examination of celebrity pregnancies and fashion trends in pregnancy sheds light on how the public situates and signifies the role of pregnancy in culture.

Chapter seven explores the commoditization of pregnancy. Marshall McLuhan argued that when people extend their sensory experience outside of their nervous system, they relinquish control of it and open it up for commoditization.[3] Today, pregnancy has emerged as another demographic, and the fetus is the newest target market. Companies use data mining to find and sell to pregnant women. Cradle-to-grave marketing strategies have extended to the womb. Pregnancy is the latest subject for reality television, as celebrities show off their bellies and use their status to sell products and services to the pregnant market. As more people become involved in the pregnant experience, new conflicts in the workplace and the law emerge over who controls what happens in the womb.

This book delves into spaces where pregnancy has become visible: You-Tube, blogs, television, fashion shows, books, film, photography, and advertisements are a few of these places. I spoke with pregnant women and expectant dads about the changes they have experienced during pregnancy.[4] I also have consulted with those who are integrated into the lives of pregnant women: friends, family, doctors, and medical technicians. I examined the cultural products marketed to pregnant women and the public at large, from pregnancy tests to photo frames for your first sonogram. It is my hope that this holistic method presents a map of the pregnant experience today and contextualizes that experience within historical and cultural frameworks.

Throughout this book, a historical context helps to understand trends in pregnancy and separate new from recurring phenomena. The home birth movement, as promoted in Ricky Lake's film *The Business of Being Born,* takes on new significance when viewed as the latest turn of a cycle from home to hospital and back. A historical perspective also illuminates the unintended consequences of pregnancy technology: though doctors use medical tests and equipment to ensure the safety of the fetus, they also have created anxiety among pregnant women, despite evidence demonstrating a birth survival rate that has grown over the last century. One hundred years ago, women would prepare sincerely for the possibility that they may not survive birth and someone else would have to raise their child. Women today are less anxious about their own survival than about all the possibilities of something going wrong with their fetus.

I detail how marketers are capitalizing on this fear by inventing products and services for pregnant women, as well as for expectant dads. I also demonstrate how the commoditization of pregnancy has allowed it to become a lifestyle and social symbol so that anyone, pregnant or not, can participate. This shift in the representation of pregnancy creates new issues to consider, from the effects of glamorizing pregnancy to the new political power of the fetus. On a more practical level, this book may help pregnant couples reconsider which products they need or want. Ultimately, the goal of this book is to examine what is gained, and what is lost, when technology and electronic media transform the pregnant experience.

Chapter 2

A Window into the Womb

One hundred years ago, a stork that swooped down to deliver a little bundle of joy was the dominant image associated with pregnancy and birth. The stork, long a part of birthing mythology because of its instinct for monogamous mating, allowed polite society to conceal the mechanics of conception while allowing family and friends to celebrate the ultimate consequence of pregnancy: the birth. While it continues to be a popular baby shower decoration, the euphemism of the stork delivering a baby is no longer necessary, for a baby has "arrived" long before its birth. Today, parents-to-be are creating Facebook pages for their unborn children, complete with a sonogram as the profile picture.[1] Images of the developing fetus via ultrasound are readily displayed on television, through e-mail, in advertisements, and by family members. The fetal image has entered the public consciousness and become reified so that, even for a pregnant woman looking at an image of her own child, one forgets that the image is mediated. In fact, the image can be produced only through the use of advanced photographic and radiology equipment, which shapes the context in which the image is produced and received. This chapter looks back to how women and the public understood or imagined the fetus prior to ultrasound technology. Then, tracing the history of the development of modern ultrasound equipment, the chapter explores how the use of this technology changes our understanding of and relationship to the fetus and pregnancy.

Imagining Pregnancy

Before the common use of imaging technologies and medical testing, women only had their imaginations, myths or traditions, and senses to allow them connect and bond with their fetus, as well as predict how it will develop as their child. In her research on the history of birth, Tina Cassidy summarizes that from the beginning, women have relied on "wives tales, icons, and rituals to make sense of pregnancy and birth, to determine everything from the baby's sex to its due date."[2] She cites examples such as midwives burning frankincense, giving pregnant women beads or idols to hold, and prompting them to utter chants and drink potions.[3] Prior to the development of modern technology, the treatment of pregnancy was a guessing game.

One routine purpose of performing an ultrasound today is to help determine the date of conception. Prior to this procedure, doctors could only guess at the gestation period for humans. Ancient scholars like Aristotle, Hippocrates, and Pythagoras offered their own theories on how to estimate durations of pregnancy. Hippocrates, for example, tried to date a pregnancy based on the first movement of the fetus.[4]

Despite their prevalence, fertility rites were not discussed openly in Western culture prior to the 19th century. The Catholic Church, in its efforts to discourage fertility rites, actively suppressed information about them.[5] During the 17th century, many women found it difficult to determine whether they were pregnant. Jacques Gélis, a French scholar on birth and midwifery, explored early theories of pregnancy in his book *History of Childbirth: Fertility, Pregnancy, and Birth in Early Modern Europe.* He writes, "Signs of pregnancy might sometimes be so ambiguous or hard to interpret that a woman was wrongly believed to be pregnant when she was not, while an actual pregnancy was not discovered until it was quite well advanced."[6]

In part because pregnancy was such a private, mysterious affair, the mother played a more pronounced role in the nourishment of the fetus than today. Although women now are admonished to rest and watch what they eat for the health of the fetus, prior to this modern period, even the mother's thoughts and imaginations about the fetus were thought to influence fetal development. Ancient Hindu medical treatises warned that mothers should satisfy their longings because that was how the fetus expressed its wishes.[7] A theory of maternal impressions emerged during the Renaissance in which the importance of the magical relationship of the mother and fetus was stressed by comparing that relationship to the unity of the world.[8] A book for pregnant women written in 1671 warns that a common cause of women's miscarriage "is their longings, and sometimes of their unnatural and unreasonable desires after they have conceived with Child: You must know, that to exceed in the things not natural as Philosophers call eating and drinking, fullness, emptiness, sleep and watchings, exercise and rest, and too great intention of the mind, may hasten the birth, and cause abortion."[9] A pregnant woman not only had to watch what she ate, but also what she thought, lest her baby be adversely affected. Likewise, birthmarks were thought to be evidence of unsatisfied urges. Some beliefs that seem absurd today were held as gospel at the time, including: "The mother's craving for milk could lead to a white strip of hair, a mother's fear of pigs could lead to a cleft palate, her stepping on the hair thrown out the window by a barber could lead to an abnormally hairy child, and so on."[10]

It was not just a matter of what women thought, but also what they did. Women were advised to avoid disturbing experiences and romantic novels "that filled their heads—and presumably the fetus's mind—with trivial ideas, but also to abstain from serious study, which might draw vital blood from the uterus to the brain, limiting fetal growth."[11] Even once the early medical practitioners, male midwives called accoucheurs, no longer believed in the direct link between what a woman imagined and the connection to the fetus, women were still warned to avoid undue emotion during pregnancy. The fear of the responsibility that rests in pregnant women is a theme in early writing, such as Mary Wollstonecraft's *A Vindication of the Rights of Women.*[12]

Everyday women were not the only ones who heeded these warnings—medical journals reported many of these stories as fact. Although this theory waned among intellectuals during the 19th century, it continued to persist within the popular imagination and managed to find its way into some literary and scientific texts.[13] An 1842 advice book illustrates an attempt by the author to refute these beliefs for mothers.[14] Yet, these myths were difficult to dispel. In the 1940s and 1950s, psychologists developed the field of prenatal psychology. Prior to the 20th century, philosophers and medical practitioners imagined an important connection between the mind of the pregnant woman and the health of her fetus. Psychologists attempted to formalize these notions by treating women who suffered physical symptoms of unknown cause with psychoanalysis.[15] A 1957 advice book indicates that these myths continued to persist: "Many a young woman, with commendable determination, has set her facial muscles into a constant grin for nine long months because certain well-intentioned elders have told her that a cheerful attitude on her part ensured a cheerful disposition in her offspring."[16]

In addition to being careful about what she imagined, a woman's senses were important in the developing pregnancy. A key moment between mother and fetus was the sense of touch—quickening—the point in the pregnancy when women could first feel movement. As other scholars have previously explored,[17] this is a significant moment because it is a mother's chance to formulate a special bond with her baby. This knowledge is hers alone as she is the only one to physically experience the moment.

Gélis describes the eye as "the mirror of the pregnancy."[18] Since women were the only ones in touch with their pregnancy, people would look in their eyes to determine if they were pregnant. Prior to the widespread use of imaging technology, doctors could treat pregnant women based on only what they could observe themselves, forcing them to rely on women as the primary medium to examine the fetus. Women were in the privileged position of knowing the most intimate details of their pregnancy. Now, visualization technologies have replaced the eye as the window into the womb. The development of imaging technology threatens this exclusive bond between mother and child. Although premodern conceptions of pregnancy may have overplayed the role of the mother in influencing the health of her fetus, the current view encourages women to rely on technology at the expense of their own senses and induces them to distrust their instincts. As we examine the growth of technology that peers into the womb, a paradox that emerges is the ability of the mother to visually bond with her child while subsuming her tactile sensory connection to the fetus.

Predicting Pregnancy

Attempts to test for pregnancy date back to as early as Ancient Greece. Aristotle had advised straining urine and looking for living creatures in the remains. In 1350 BC, Egyptian pregnant women could conduct a wheat test: a woman's urine was used to water the wheat and see if the wheat grew, under the assumption that the hormones in the urine could germinate seeds. In the 13th century, Magnus had created a milk test: milk was mixed with urine; if the milk floated above the urine, the woman was pregnant.[19]

Although these tests were not always conclusive and often misleading, determining if one was pregnant was, for many women, a solitary experience that involved getting in touch with their own bodies. Doctors, midwives, and others had to rely on a mother's account to make any kind of diagnosis. A 17th-century book for midwives advises to look to the mother for signs of pregnancy, such as unusual actions on her part: "She hath a preternatural desire to something not fit to eat nor drink, as some women with child have longed to bite off a piece of their Husband's Buttocks."[20] Other signs might include loss of her "monthly terms" and a weak stomach, but those these physical symptoms were considered to be less reliable. A book for midwives written over two centuries later still discusses the difficulty in making a correct diagnosis: "Apart from the patches of pigmented skin which are occasionally seen, a woman's face often gives, especially to one who knows it, indications of pregnancy. This, however, is of much less value than the complaint of 'morning sickness.' This may be merely a feeling of nausea'soon after rising, or a complete or partial vomiting of the morning meal, the nausea soon passing off."[21] The author goes on to suggest that the movement of the fetus can also be another reliable method. Less reliable is the lack of menstruation "because the fear of being pregnant may lead woman to have a loss of menses."[22] The common element of these indicators is that they all are intimately connected to the mother and her senses; she alone stands as the mediator between the fetus and the outside world.

In 1928, the hormone progesterone was identified, allowing for the development of the Aschheim-Zondek (A-Z) test, the first pregnancy test for women. This test involved injecting mice with a woman's urine. After being incubated for 100 hours, the mice were killed and their ovaries inspected. If the organs were enlarged and congested, the woman was pregnant. Later, rabbits were substituted in place of mice, creating the culturally popular expression "rabbit test."[23] By the 1960s, new tests that no longer required animals allowed doctors to administer the tests in their offices.[24] As pregnancy testing transformed from an observational activity in the home to a technology-laden scientific enterprise, the discovery of pregnancy became the privilege of medical professionals. A woman might suspect she was pregnant, but the doctor was the first to know. Thus began the deterioration of pregnancy as the exclusive domain of the mother, for she was no longer the most reliable source for this discovery.

The home pregnancy test, approved by the FDA in 1977, represents the next significant advance in pregnancy testing.[25] Soon after its approval, advertisements for the new test appeared in women's magazines. For just $10, women could find out in the privacy of their own homes whether they were pregnant. Sarah Leavitt has studied the history of the pregnancy test for the National Institutes of Health. She describes how early advertisements "wavered between an emphasis on science and a more emotional appeal." Leavitt's study reports the challenge of marketing a test where women, in isolation, would discover a result that would be joyful for some and upsetting for others.[26]

The ability of women to test themselves at home granted them an unprecedented privacy in finding out potentially life-changing news. In some sense, it allowed for women to have the potential to retain their own perhaps ambivalent feelings about the result. With a doctor's office, they are expected to put on a show and a smile and act happy. With a test, one is entitled to one's personal feelings. During my interviews with pregnant women, many have confided that, after an initial moment of elation upon finding out they were pregnant, they then cried out of fear. Even women who were desperate to get pregnant experienced conflicting emotions when they discovered they achieved their goal. These home tests allow women complete confidentiality, and they have the power of choosing when, or if, to reveal their news. In this case, technology restores some power to women, who once again could choose to be the only one to know about their pregnancy.

However, unlike pregnancy during the pretechnological era, home pregnancy tests press women to trust technology over their own senses. My own experience illustrates this point. When I thought I was pregnant with my first child, I purchased a digital pregnancy test. The test indicated a positive result by displaying the word "pregnant." When I saw the word appear, I felt excited and showed it to my husband. We then left the test in our bathroom as we telephoned my family to tell them the news. Later, I returned to the bathroom and picked up the test. The display was blank. I knew that results on some home tests fade or disappear with time, and I knew on a rational level that I was pregnant, but part of me was upset that the words disappeared. The scientific validation of my pregnancy was gone. I suddenly had an overwhelming urge to purchase another test immediately to regain the certain, authoritative pronouncement of my pregnancy.

My feelings illustrate what these tests have done. Before, women relied on their senses to intuit that they were pregnant. They then waited for a physical, natural symptom, such as the absence of menses or a growing abdomen, to confirm what they felt. Today, an external test provides prompt notification. Manufacturers of these tests often sell them in packages of two or three. Apparently, they expect women to not be satisfied with the result of one test, so they include a second one for the reassurance of a "second opinion." Of course, for many women attempting to conceive, the process often requires many months and many tests, and some women may test too early and receive a false negative the first time. Regardless, a second test is comforting to have.

Pregnancy tests increasingly are marketing themselves as early predictors. Just the title of the "First Response" pregnancy test makes almost unnecessary its tagline, "Being there FIRST for women."[27] EPT describes itself as the "error proof test" and claims that a woman can test up to four days prior to her period.[28] Yet, testing early brings new problems along with solutions. When the tests were first created, one of the challenges that marketers had to confront was the stigma attached with early knowledge: for many, wanting early pregnancy notification was a sign of promiscuity.[29]

Today, most women simply assume that, because they can have early knowledge, they should. For some, this knowledge could be useful, particularly if they want to terminate the pregnancy. Others assert that, the earlier they know, the better they can adapt their diet and lifestyle to nourish and protect their child. Some women with irregular menstrual cycles can use the test to confirm what they may have suspected but have been uncertain about for some time.

However, for the majority of women, these early tests obsolesce nature. First Response promises results "five days sooner." The test, in some ways, has created a market for news that may not be necessary; after all, women would eventually discover their pregnancy naturally, which would allow them some time to digest the news. Before testing, a gradual process gently clued women in to their pregnancy. With immediate and accurate tests, the news suddenly appears, and some women may not be ready to face it.

Testing early and bonding to the fetus often produces more of an emotional strain if the pregnancy fails. Before testing, a woman who miscarried may have never known she was pregnant. Now, a positive test result sets up attachments and expectations that may be shattered with the ending of that pregnancy. Leavitt describes how early pregnancy tests have made the miscarriage more of a community event, as more women have already told others about their pregnancies as confirmed by the test.[30] For some, this means more supporters mourn with the woman for her loss, but others may be pained by having to publicly share their sorrow.

The ubiquity of pregnancy tests has led to an online community that fetishizes the test and agonizes over the period of time when women are waiting to find out if they are pregnant. Once a solitary experience, women now can look to websites such as Peeonastick.com to analyze in detail their pregnancy test and look at images of strangers' tests submitted to the website.[31] The website TwoWeekWAIT.com offers a supportive online community to help women during the waiting period between conception and a missed period that would indicate pregnancy. They advertise, "We'll help you decide if you're pregnant. Sure, some people just take a pregnancy test and call it done (suckers, I say). Real ladies, though, like to air their symptoms to a jury of their peers to decide if they're pregnant. Scientifically valid? Maybe not. Therapeutic? Definitely!"[32] The website offers ovulation kits, fertility aids, and pregnancy tests for sale, of course. Struggling over waiting two weeks would seem inconceivable to women of previous generations, for whom waiting was both a necessary and natural process.

Manufacturers of these at-home tests market them as giving power to women. Before women could test themselves, they were dependent upon their doctors, who sometimes denied or delayed testing to preclude their patients from seeking abortions.[33] The test indeed puts knowledge in the hands of women, yet it also has the potential to take away power, too. For instance, women in Mexico are routinely punished for their pregnancies. Businesses do not want to pay government-mandated payments for maternity leave, so they force women to take pregnancy tests. Often, they justify these tests by arguing that they are seeking to shield pregnant women from dangerous work. As a result of public outcry, Rosario Robles, the mayor of Mexico City, was forced in 2000 to prohibit businesses from requiring these tests.[34] Here, a test designed to offer women more control over their lives is used to restrict their choices.

As with all commercial goods, once a product has saturated the marketplace, manufacturers look for innovative ways to market their brand. The pregnancy test has followed pregnancy itself in becoming a more open, accepted, and even celebrated part of culture. Advertisers have capitalized on this by launching campaigns that promote pregnancy testing as a common, casual experience. Clearblue Easy created an advertisement where urinating is the primary hook. The voice over narrator intones, "Introducing the most sophisticated piece of technology . . . you will ever pee on." The director of the ad campaign said that internally they were calling it "the pregnancy test for the *Sex and the City* generation."[35] Pregnancy testing is marketed to a culture that considers itself sexually savvy,[36] and tests even have been used to promote other products. One book publisher had a character in a bath so engrossed in a new book that she was oblivious to the results of the pregnancy test she had just taken.[37] The pregnancy test, designed to offer women privacy, is no longer a private affair. In fact, the pregnancy test itself has become an artifact to preserve. Women now save their pregnancy tests to include in their child's baby memory book. Some even post pictures of their urine-filled tests on their blogs or websites. The home test has become another aspect of pregnancy that has shifted from the private to the public sphere.

Making Pregnancy Portable

Another major change in modern pregnancy is the ultrasound. Its introduction has redefined the relationship of the mother to the fetus and pregnancy to the outside world. Prior to the invention of this technology, little was known about the developing fetus. Doctors had to rely on a mother's senses to diagnose the health of her baby.[38] In the 19th century, as male doctors began to care for pregnant women, conducting a more thorough examination conflicted with the social mores of Victorian society. Doctors had to persuade women it was acceptable and necessary to allow them to conduct internal exams in an age when the stethoscope was rejected as indecent.[39] To protect the privacy of the mother, doctors often conducted exams with women facing away from them to avoid eye contact.[40] Ultimately, however, technology provided a window into the world of the fetus and, by association, its mother.

Prior to the invention of the ultrasound, doctors used models and drawings to explain reproductive anatomy to other doctors and professionals in the field. Deborah L. Spar in her book *The Baby Business: How Money, Science, and Politics Drive the Commerce of Conception* provides an example in 1844 of Frederick Hollick, a doctor who used "life-sized papier-mâché models. Hollick gave his audiences a complete tour of human anatomy, including, he boasted, 'the development of the new being in the womb at every stage.'"[41] The first pictures of the womb emerged thanks to Wilhelm Rontgen's invention of the X-ray in 1895.[42] However, this method was less than desirable because the extra fat and amniotic fluid reduced the resolution of the image.[43]

The development of the technology allowing us to finally peer into the womb was actually an effort in warfare. British engineers worked on sonar technology to fight the Axis powers during World War I. Over 30 years passed before a Scottish medical scientist, Ian Donald, used sonar to see a fetus in gestation. Ultrasound technology was significant because it allowed doctors to examine the fetus in unprecedented detail in a way that did not involve physically invading a woman's body. Most gynecologists in Europe and United States were using ultrasound machines within a decade of their introduction in 1962. Prior to the late 1970s, ultrasounds produced low-resolution images that showed mostly a fetus's bone tissue. Later, scan converters made for better pictures, and advances in video technology allowed people to see the surface features of the fetus.[44]

Parents who proudly show sonograms of their future child have *Life* magazine to thank for setting this precedent. In its April 30, 1965, issue, photographer Lennart Nilsson published his pictures of a fetus inside a womb.[45] For the first time, the American public was able to see in full color on a prominent magazine cover what before could only be imagined. During this same period, theorist Marshall McLuhan observed that media employ the power to extend one's senses. From this point forward, doctors would use ultrasounds for more than merely medical purposes; the imaging extends the pregnancy experience to others and enhances the ability of the mother to not only feel her fetus from within, but to also see it exposed.

Jose van Dijck, a scholar at the University of Amsterdam, is the leading expert on the cultural impact of visual imaging technology. In her extensive work on this subject, she has explored the disparity between the intentions of the creators of the technology and the unexpected results of it. She writes that real-time video was intended for scientists to conduct comparative research on fetuses, but doctors found that women wanted to see their babies: "Women loved seeing images of their fetuses moving around in the uterus, on the screen, even if they were quite incapable of interpreting them correctly."[46]

In the 1980s, scientists began studies to measure the effectiveness of fetal ultrasounds on parental bonding. While ultrasounds often look alike, women were now encouraged to see them as personalized.[47] By 1985, ultrasounds became a standard practice during prenatal exams.[48] Although the terms are sometimes used interchangeably, the ultrasound refers to the technology, while the sonogram refers to the picture that is produced as a result of the technology. Today, the sonogram image has become ubiquitous. Routinely, technicians give women high-quality pictures to take home with them, and some take home videos of their babies. Doctors post pictures of their patients' fetuses on the walls of their waiting rooms. Women e-mail pictures of their womb to their friends and family members. The accessibility of the sonogram allows it to become a common point of reference for the pregnancy experience.

The previous chapter mapped pregnancy as it moved from a social experience with other women in the mother's community to a medical experience, and eventually to a combined social/medical experience. Here, the transformation reverses: pregnancy moves from a medical experience to a social one, eventually settling to a combined social/medical experience. Women whom I have interviewed about their ultrasound experience illustrate how technology alters the social dynamics of pregnancy.

A woman in New York City, Mary,[49] talks about her doctor's love of ultrasounds: "My doctor is ultrasound crazy. He has a small machine that he uses to check the heartbeat and position every time you are there." Yet, she describes her frustration with her sonograms: "I felt like it was a bit of a violation to show the ultrasound pictures, especially to my parents. I wasn't planning to be pregnant so I wanted to keep it to myself. I didn't really want to share. Whereas my husband was e-mailing the pictures to the whole family and I was kind of getting annoyed." For some, an ultrasound can result in psychological benefits because it allows for reassurance and bonding.[50] For Mary, though, the pictures from the ultrasound resulted in her pregnancy being made public earlier than she would have liked.[51] Like pregnancy before testing, the ultrasound disrupts a woman's natural right for private time to adjust to the idea of having a baby.

Janelle Taylor has written extensively on the social effects of the modern ultrasound. As the experience became less a purely medical one, the physical space in which the ultrasound took place was also transformed. Additional chairs were added to the sonogram room to allow for the accommodation of a spouse and others.[52] Today, a pregnant woman and her guests can easily see video monitors during the "examination." Ultrasounds also change the dynamic between prospective mothers and fathers, who have become producers of ultrasound documentaries. Since they no longer need to wait until the birth to become involved, the ultrasound has become a useful tool for men to process and experience what the fetus is doing. It is not uncommon for men to record the ultrasound experience, making a video of a video.

Another pregnant woman said her husband became so involved in capturing the viewing of her ultrasound for prosperity that he talked about bringing his computer to the next ultrasound in order to improve the sound quality of his recording. She observed, "It's really easy to get so subsumed with the documentary processes of having a kid that you're not entirely present." Technology allows for the father to be involved in the pregnancy, but his involvement centers on using his own media technology to capture the ultrasound, distancing him from the experience. His wife notices the irony of technology that has the potential to bring her husband closer to her experience, but instead leads him to somewhat miss it.

Taylor also discusses the changing relationship between the sonographer (more often than not, a woman) and the pregnant patient. Because the technology does not require any ionizing radiation, the sonographer can stay in the examination room, encouraging her to talk with the pregnant woman and provide her with details about her baby, such as its position, sex, or character traits.[53] During my own experience, the sonographer typed words she attributed to the fetus onto the sonogram for me to take home. Others have talked about how the sonographer described their baby as tired, cranky, active, or pretty. These attributions may encourage parents to identify with the fetus. At the same time, these comments help to generate meaning from the process. Watching an image of a floating amniotic sac may not be as fascinating if one were not providing a running commentary, but it also results in conceptualizing the fetus as a baby earlier in the pregnancy. By attributing thoughts, ideas, and actions to a fetus that could not possibly produce them, the fetus is thought of as being more advanced and as more of a person. Politically, the impact of this can be seen easily within the pro-life movement as they have incorporated posters and videos of fetuses to bolster their argument that life begins at conception. Church groups, for example, have begun offering women free sonograms in an attempt to persuade them from ending their pregnancies.[54]

On a personal level, seeing the fetus at this early stage inspires couples to bond with their baby earlier and desire even more information about their future child. In our new media environment, we have lost the notion of waiting. We live in an on-demand society, where we can order entertainment or information when we want it. Pregnancy, until now, has been one of those natural processes that force us to wait for what we want. However, the innovation of the nonmedical ultrasound allows people to have an opportunity to see their growing baby on their own time. One company called Fetal Fotos advertises "an ultrasound experience to treasure for a lifetime." The business promises the latest technology "to help parents bond with their baby."[55] It allows women a virtually unlimited amount of time to view their fetus. Instead of medical professionals guiding the process, parents can find out the answers to their own questions, ranging from facial features to the sex of the baby.

While ultrasound technology originally was employed to diagnose medical conditions, the technology now mimics the language of film for the purpose of entertainment. Some facilities produce a DVD for parents, allowing them to choose music to accompany the moving images. A quick search of YouTube using the keywords "baby ultrasound" yields over 2,000 hits. Some make political statements, but most are just parents showing off their babies-to-be, synced to their favorite music. As evidence that we have immersed ourselves in an MTV culture, babies can now star in their first music video, straight from the womb.

Inventors of ultrasound technology borrowed ideas from media technology, like film, which allows people to not only record images of reality but also to manipulate them, or create images from scratch. J. van Dijck recognizes the important connections between media and medical technologies. She writes:

> Between the early fifteenth and the early twenty-first century, a plethora of visual and representational instruments have been developed to help obtain new views on, and convey new insights into human physiology. From the pen of the anatomical illustrator to the surgeon's advanced endoscopic techniques, instruments of visualization and observation have mediated our perceptions of the interior body through an intricate mixture of scientific investigation, artistic observation, and public understanding.[56]

This early relationship between aesthetic visual technologies and medical visualization has reversed into a confusing world of "medictainment" as the medical and entertainment worlds have blended in an experience in which the ultrasound is packaged as entertainment. Consumer products, like picture frames for a sonogram, are now made for parents to display the image of their fetus for others.

The ultrasound has even become a focal point for television commercials.[57] A GE ad for an ultrasound system plays the song "The First Time Ever I Saw Your Face" while showing parents looking at a very clear image of a baby with its mouth moving. The narrator intones, "When you see your baby for the first time on the GE 4D Ultrasound System, it really is a miracle," as the husband and wife caress their hands on her belly. A dissolve from the ultrasound to the parents lying with their newborn baby collapses the time from that first image to after birth and fuses the material world with an image of that world.

A music video of Massive Attack's song "Teardrop" consists of the moving image of a fetus in the womb. The video alternates viewpoints between the baby in the womb and the world from the fetus's perspective. The baby is supposedly lip-synching the music. This video uses extreme close-up shots to show parts of the body such as the baby's eye or its hands touching its mouth. Also prominent is the umbilical cord, emphasizing the connection of the baby to a mother we never see. Clearly, the fetus is the star of this video. On the website Answerbag.com, fans of the video debate its meaning, ranging from the fetus being a metaphor for human beings as empty slates ready for the world or a love song from a mother to a child, to another fan who thinks the video means to be an antiabortion testimony.[58] While the meaning is certainly open for interpretation, what is significant is that the fetus plays a role just like any actor.

The conflation of the ultrasound with a future baby is used by performers such as Nick Cannon to put forward a pro-life message. Cannon claims that his song "Can I Live" is a true story about his mother's decision not to abort him when she was pregnant as a teenager. He sings like an angel from the future, pleading with his mother to not go through with the abortion she was considering. Just before the procedure, the angelic Cannon places his hands on his mother's belly while the ultrasound monitor shows the fetus. He sings, "What is becoming, ma, I am Oprah-bound. You can tell he's a star from the ultrasound." The future life of this fetus is projected onto this ultrasound moment.

You do not need to be a musician to create a music video of your baby-to-be. Parents now routinely post their sonogram videos up on YouTube to show off their expectant families. Sometimes they are left as is with the doctor's voice in the background. But, more often than not, they are set to music, so each baby is starring in its own amateur music video. Relatives of the couple are then free to comment about the baby, especially how cute it looks. The ubiquitous ultrasound video being used for entertainment illustrates the lack of privacy connected to the womb. The ultrasound music video is replacing the baby portrait as the baby's first photo-shoot.

Currently, the cost of an ultrasound device and the skill required to operate it stand in the way of people who want to purchase their own machines for private viewing. There are exceptions, however. When Tom Cruise's then-girlfriend Katie Holmes became pregnant, Cruise purchased an ultrasound machine for their home. *People* magazine quoted Cruise regarding Holmes's ultrasound: "The sonogram was fun, though. Those pictures you can get are incredible. I'm a filmmaker—I need to see the rushes!"[59] Cruise, perhaps one of Hollywood's most recognizable stars, equates the sonogram to what he knows: a preview of his film. However, rushes are works in progress, expected to be edited and adapted by the filmmakers. In the past, babies developed on their own with minimal interference from events happening outside the womb. Cruise's comments reflect the reconceptualization that this technology enables.

The ultrasound has the power to change the relationship between not only the mother and father or the mother and the fetus, but also the fetus and the outside world. Views differ regarding the benefits and drawbacks to the ultrasound. While some argue that it reassures and promotes parental bonding, others charge that it creates a nervous, apprehensive attitude for which a fetus must pass certain tests.[60] Still others worry about unknown medical side effects. The FDA has issued warnings about entertainment ultrasounds. In New York, a legislator is attempting to introduce legislation to ban the practice.[61] One consequence that receives much less attention is that, concurrently with the creation of technology that peers in at the fetus, new technologies allow parents to stimulate the fetus.[62] As parents peek in for a view, the consequential next step is the attempt to interact with the fetus.

Fetal Testing: Peering in, Finding Out

In the past, parents were forced to wait over nine months during pregnancy before seeing their baby, but now, within a culture of immediate gratification, they can begin to see the fetus practically from conception. The ability to peer in prior to birth also leads to the desire to interact with the fetus. This involvement can take a number of forms.

More prospective parents are using some form of prenatal screening to test their newborn for a variety of conditions. This technology was first created to diagnose serious illnesses for which there were, at the time, no real treatments.[63] More advanced research has led to tests that screen much earlier in the pregnancy. One such test allows for first trimester screening for diseases such as Down syndrome.[64] A new test under development can map the genome of a fetus with blood from the mother and saliva from the expectant father.[65] For some, the prenatal screening is a blessing, as surgery can cure many conditions. Parents may choose to abort a fetus that would otherwise be born with birth defects. Others see the screening as a burden. These tests consume some women during their first trimester with the fear that they will reveal something wrong with the fetus.[66]

With fetal testing come new lawsuits in the area of reproductive law. Sometimes couples will sue when prenatal testing does not reveal birth defects that later emerge. A *New York Times* article profiled couples who were upset that the medical establishment had not provided them with enough information about their unborn children.[67] Some couples are using new tests to determine what diseases their future child could possibly inherit, allowing them to weed out undesired embryos. Parents are screening now for colon and breast cancer, but there is some debate over what this technology, called pre-implantation genetic diagnosis, could be used for in the future.[68] Does extensive testing bias people toward abortion, encouraging a modern version of eugenics? Others worry that prenatal testing could lead to parents preselecting a more intelligent child, or the creation of a fetal test for homosexuality.[69] A controversial product that generated much press was the Baby Gender Mentor, marketed by the company Acu-Gen as having the ability to determine the sex of a baby very early in the pregnancy.[70] The product, which costs $275, tests the mother's blood. Parents have claimed that the tests are faulty, but the company stands by its product, explaining away erroneous results as the detection of a "vanishing twin."[71] The concept of women testing their fetuses at home follows the path of pregnancy testing itself. The at-home pregnancy test created both freedoms and constraints. In the same way, fetal testing at home allows parents to control information and their decisions about what to do with it. At the same time, when the fetus is examined in this way, it becomes a commodity, separated from the mother as the parents may choose whether they want to accept certain characteristics attached to it.

As a fetus's traits are examined, the next logical step for parents is to begin communicating with it during the pregnancy. It used to be that mothers had to wait for the fetus to interact with her before she was truly aware of its existence. Before that point, there was no way to know that the baby was responding in some way to outside stimuli. This was known traditionally as the quickening stage, when the mother would feel the first kick. With modern technology, this is no longer a one-way relationship. Parents don't wait for the baby to announce its presence; instead, they make early attempts to communicate with the fetus. Mothers have, of course, always talked to their pregnant bellies, and fathers used this method as a way to experience the pregnancy. However, parents increasingly are using more advanced technology as the mediator between themselves and their fetus. Some parents have played music in the hopes that it might inspire a budding Mozart or Beethoven. It is one thing to listen to music in the hope that the baby will absorb some of it. In fact, this takes us back to the early maternal myths that the thoughts and actions of the mother will impact her fetus. Yet, the next step, putting headphones on your belly so that the baby directly will benefit from this music, takes the mother out of the equation. In the second scenario, one acknowledges that the fetus exists as a separate identity entitled to its own stimulation, education, and entertainment.

Prior to fetal stimulation technologies, women simply played music for their baby. Now, they can use products such as the BabyPlus prenatal education system. The BabyPlus system describes itself as mental nourishment for the fetus: "Much like a prenatal vitamin enriches the nutritional environment of a child during pregnancy, our curriculum enriches the auditory environment." The product uses an audio device that introduces patterns of sound similar to the mother's heartbeat. The manufacturer claims, "As a baby discriminates the heartbeat sounds of BabyPlus from those of the mother, learning has begun and the child's brain has been activated in a way never before possible."[72] One set of parents I interviewed said that this audio device video allowed them to "jump start learning." The mother thought of the technology as a way to begin teaching her baby even before it was born. In an age when the competition for a quality education is so intense, mothers feel pressured to begin their child's education at an earlier age. Now, mothers can begin this process even before their child's birth. Additionally, it gives the husband some empowerment during the pregnancy. In our interview, the prospective father said, "At least I can contribute in some way besides biologically." Like ultrasound technology, this software brings the father into the process earlier.

"Make Way for Baby!" is another fetal stimulation tool advertised online. It describes itself as taking an "interactive approach to prenatal stimulation," based on scientific research from scholars studying the impact of prenatal stimulation.[73] Rather than simply pipe prerecorded sounds to the fetus, the video encourages parents to create their own stimulation exercises that follow given examples. Once a baby is born, other products promise parents to replicate the experience in the womb. These technologies reinforce the notion that a fetus is extremely aware of and comforted by the unique experience in the womb, and that a baby remembers this experience. Some parents swear by these devices, while others find them useless, but these products bring into clear focus that the fetus is now seen differently than it has been in the past. The fetus is becoming more and more its own entity in the womb, separate from its mother. Pamela Paul, in her book *Parenting Inc.*, discusses the popularity of prenatal educational software. Paul notes the global reach of this market, describing BabyPlus as "growing between 15 percent and 25 percent each year, and in 2006, it sold about eight thousand devices in sixty countries worldwide."[74] This enables the transformation of the fetus into a commodity, as products are marketed toward its development and comfort, which creates a number of political, social, and economic ramifications as examined later in this book.

The Birth

In times past, birth was a significant moment beyond simply marking the end of the pregnancy. It was the moment in which the baby became its own person. Others could interact with the new being, who previously was hidden within its mother. Now, with the increased use of educational, photographic, and other media technologies prior to birth, this moment is becoming less significant as a defining moment when parents and their baby meet, for they already have been communicating, seeing, and learning about their new charge.

Before the 20th century, childbirth was not up for public discussion. There was little mention of it in fiction; what accounts exist are hidden within the private writing of women or in anonymous letters written to magazines.[75] Childbirth, though, was still a communal event for women. In late 18th-century Europe and America, it was still common for female relatives and neighbors to attend the birth.[76] Although childbirth was a shared experience for these women, it remained private and was not discussed in public. Women with specialized birthing knowledge became known as midwives.[77] In the 19th century, just as the medical profession began to oversee the care of pregnant women, private nurses become involved in the birthing process and to assist with the care of the infant afterward.[78] Despite the medicalization of birth, it remained a private moment, shielded from public view.

Gradually, friends and relatives attended births less and less. Some historians put the blame on the rising use of doctors, but others suggest that geographic mobility prevented families and friends from being together.[79] During the 19th century in Europe and North America, male medical professionals gradually displaced the midwife.[80] By the beginning of the 20th century, legislators throughout the United States outlawed midwifery, which solidified the medical profession as the primary authority for childbirth.[81]

In her book, *Birth: The Surprising History of How We are Born,* Tina Cassidy describes early maternity wards in late 19th century as "wretched places, mostly serving poor immigrants in big cities."[82] Cassidy relays stories of pregnant woman mistreated by doctors and losing their babies or dying of infections from these unclean hospitals.[83] Birthrates in hospitals surged in the 1940s because the federal government paid for the care of soldiers' wives during the war.[84] As hospitals sought to create a more sanitary environment, they instituted strict rules that ultimately made it more difficult for women to use natural childbirth methods and bond with their baby. The 1960s and 1970s ushered in the alternative childbirth movement as a way to revive traditional birthing.[85] Childbirth had thus come full circle, back to the home and midwives. Today, while some women do choose to birth at home, most give birth in hospitals that mimic the home birth experience.

Fathers have become more involved in the birthing experience as well. In 1962, Robert A. Bradley published *Father's Presence in Delivery Rooms,* which explained that women relaxed more when men were allowed into their labor rooms. Previously, doctors thought fathers brought harmful germs into the delivery room and interfered with their wife's modesty.[86] Fathers have now become a routine part of the birthing experience.

Not only do fathers routinely appear in the delivery room, but extended family also can pop in and visit. Many parents bring their younger children with them so they can watch their sibling being born. And, for those unable (or unwilling) to make it to the live event, videotaping the birth has become a common way of preserving the birth for others.

In *The Farmer and the Obstetrician,* Michel Odent offers a political motivation for the origin of the introduction of cameras in the delivery room: "To put forward pictures that showed alternatives to childbirth with the mother on a table, under bright lights, with her legs on stirrups, surrounded by several white-coated people."[87] Perhaps, the introduction of cameras did serve as propaganda for an alternative birthing movement. Yet, I would like to offer some alternative reasons for the increase of videotaping.

First, as people are able to peer into the womb and see the fetus during pregnancy, it is a natural progression to use media technology to continue viewing it as it enters the world. Videotaping the birth is simply an extension of photography used prior to birth. Second, as fathers increasingly are present at the birth, recording the delivery offers them an active role aside from simply assisting the mother.

As parents become more familiar with their fetus during pregnancy, birth loses some meaning as the boundary of the baby's introduction to its parents. These days, many parents have named their baby prior to its birth and call it by its name when talking to it or others. Perhaps videotaping the birth restores significance to the event by making it a media event. A birth photographer is a rapidly growing profession focused solely on professionally capturing the birth moment.[88]

Of course, as with all technologies, there are unintended consequences. As cameras are brought into the delivery room, the birth is turned into a spectacle. In fact, some hospitals now prohibit people from videotaping their births because of fear of malpractice suits. The Swedish Covenant Hospital in Chicago has turned down requests by parents to videotape births.[89] Doctors argue that the cameras invade their privacy, compromise the sterile environment, and distract fathers from the delivery.[90] Yet the increase use of cameras in the hospital room also has a potentially strong cultural impact. It is a common experience for women to forget many of the details of the birth right after. My mother always told me this was so that women would still have a desire to have more children. But my mother's self-imposed amnesia is lost to this generation. Whatever is forgotten will now be replayed on your home television. Will this encourage women to "look the part" when delivering? In fact, expectant mothers can now purchase special gowns to wear while giving birth. The Pretty Pushers online store offers all types of colors, including a sexy black gown that is also disposable.[91] Will doctors and nurses need to reexamine their bedside delivery practices because they are not only practicing their medical craft but also performing for the camera? Despite the Swedish Covenant Hospital's efforts to turn away cameras, it will be interesting to see how other hospitals adapt to make themselves camera friendly. It was not long ago that the ultrasound room adapted itself to accommodate family viewing of the growing fetus. The birthing room has already accommodated extended family by creating a type of home living room experience. The next stage may be making itself YouTube friendly. There is no shortage of birth videos on YouTube. In fact, you can even choose the type you prefer, such as a home birth or a water birth. One can only image a future YouTube experience where advertisers and hospitals work together to place products in exciting birth videos. One performance artist staged a public birth experience by converting a gallery space into her own birthing room, complete with an inflatable pool and rocking chair. Visitors watched her live birth as seven cameras recorded the experience.[92]

Outing Pregnancy

This chapter illustrates the paradox that, the more power women obtain to see into their womb, the more they lose control, as others have the power to also peer in and influence their baby's development. The primary medium through which to understand the fetus is no longer exclusively its mother. Before the development of this technology, women felt uneasy that male doctors invaded their privacy through the physical examination of their sexual organs. Now, one need not have an invasive medical exam to determine if one is pregnant. The irony is that visualization technologies completely expose the female body. But, represented in a mediated form, the display of internal sexual organs becomes desexualized. Once the stigma of sexuality is removed, pregnancy becomes open for everybody to share and embrace as part of our consumer culture.

The modern media environment has encouraged even medical technologies to mirror and imitate technologies associated with entertainment. The ultrasound, first invented to examine the fetus for potential medical problems, has become another entertainment experience for prospective parents. Prior to the invention of these modern visualization technologies, prospective mothers could only imagine what may be going on inside their bodies. But, now that women can readily see their fetus, their imaginations have refocused upon the internal thoughts of the fetus. Parents imagine that their fetus is absorbing every outside stimulus, and they are marketed products to stimulate their fetus. The more the fetus can be seen, the more people will see it as another work-in-progress. Sometimes, this desire is expressed as life-saving prenatal medical surgeries or attempts to influence the baby's physical development. More often, parents want their prospective babies to develop a love of music, letters, science, or numbers.

In our modern consumer culture, much time and money is spent studying children's exposure to advertising and other mediated messages. People lament over the lack of public spaces where one can escape advertising. The months prior to birth used to be a sacred space for the baby, but now, thanks to technologies that allow people to test, measure, view, influence, and modify the fetus, it has fallen within reach of marketers who offer these technologies, for a price. The fetus has become the latest target market.

Mothers, the medium between the fetus and the outside world, face new questions and anxieties as the public becomes more interested in the fetus. The potential power that expectant moms have over the development of their fetus always has been scrutinized. In earlier periods, the imagination of women was thought to influence their fetus. Later, the anxiety of women was treated as a mental illness. The focus on the psyche of pregnant women manifests itself today in how the public worries about the physical and mental environment of pregnant women. The recent book *Origins: How the Nine Months before Birth Shape the Rest of Our Lives* illustrates a 21st-century interest in assessing how our fetal time influences who we become.[93] Today, we are less interested in psychoanalyzing pregnant women but are quick to warn them about how they may hurt their fetus through their lifestyle choices. New studies come out regularly that connect a pregnant woman's food choices to the weight of her baby, her exposure to fever and disorders in the fetus, and stress levels to fetal development. Pregnant women are left to worry about how they are adversely impacting their fetus, even in ways that they cannot possibly control. This interest has created new growth in an advice market ready to answer these questions and sell products as a solution to problems.

Chapter 3

It Takes an E-Village

Jenny McCarthy's book about her pregnancy is read by women who are not even thinking of becoming pregnant themselves. A video of a man filming his wife's growing pregnant belly becomes one of the most viewed videos on Google and YouTube.[1] A pregnant woman who experiences an odd symptom turns on her computer instead of calling her doctor. Women don't have to wait for their first doctor's visit to find out their estimated due date; rather, they can go to a website that calculates the exact date. All of these examples are possible because of a shift in how pregnancy is viewed within popular culture.

This chapter traces the history of pregnancy advice sharing and explores the ways in which women have received and sought out advice throughout their pregnancies. By doing so, it shows how new media environments have changed access to information about pregnancy. Industrialization and its promotion of mass production, the growth of the publishing industry, and the creation of the Internet all have played a part in this evolution. Information for this chapter has been derived from historical works, early and current advice books, blogs, discussion boards and chat rooms of pregnant women, and conversations with pregnant women who are using emerging modes of media to share their pregnancies.

Announcing Pregnancy

Once a woman finds out she is pregnant, one of the first decisions she makes is who to tell and when. Even today, many women choose not to share their early pregnancies with those outside their immediate family, and sometimes not even with anyone other than their spouse or doctor. Others, however, tell all. In the past, women were much less likely to proclaim their pregnancy. In ancient Rome, women would wear bandeaux around their necks. When the snug-fitting bands became too tight, women would take them off, and the household could celebrate.[2] We see here that the announcement is physically associated with the pregnancy: these women would make their pregnancy public when it could no longer be hidden.

Scholars find little information about the everyday lives of pregnant women before the 19th century. In fact, women were discreet, and sometimes ashamed, regarding their condition, and made efforts to conceal their pregnancies.[3] A clergyman's advice book for pregnant women in the early 19th century discusses the loneliness of the mother: "There is a bitterness which the heart of a mother alone can know, but which she cannot fully express; a class of feelings and impressions so peculiar, that will admit only of a partial and imperfect development."[4] This quote reveals the solitude of pregnant women who were encouraged to keep their feelings about their current state to themselves. Pregnancy was not a widely discussed topic during this period, even within contemporary literature.[5] To be sure, some women may have taken advantage of pregnancy to avoid social interaction, but during the mid-19th century, women began to guard pregnancy and restrict public activities out of concern for gentility. Women would remain confined during pregnancy in part to conform to the ideal standard of a social class, but a declining birthrate also allowed more women to be cautious during pregnancy.[6] While for most, pregnancy during this period was considered a private experience, some women had the luxury of making the experience a particularly comfortable one.

Communal Advice and Support: A Woman's Inner Circle

Although pregnancy was hidden, women were not without support. In 17th-century colonial America, relatives and friends commonly traveled great distances to help the pregnant woman with her household duties.[7] Jacques Gélis, a French scholar on birth and midwifery, describes pregnancy as a collective experience, as a town or village would support a number of pregnant women at any one time.[8] Yet, in the late 18th and early 19th centuries, more people left the countryside for more anonymous towns and cities. Moving away from families and friends cut women off from the traditional support of their family.[9] Thus, pregnancy support became tied closely to location and space. One needed to be physically close to people in order to receive their guidance. As people moved away, mediated communication replaced the advice initially offered directly by friends and friends. The particular characteristics of each mediated technology, such as the isolation of reading or the way the Internet encourages a specific type of interaction, shapes the advice received.

Professional Advice: From Communal
Gestation to Medical Diagnosis

The pregnancy information environment began to shift as pregnancy advice from the medical profession displaced informal pregnancy advice from family and friends. During the Middle Ages, obstetrical literature was almost nonexistent.[10] Men paid little interest in obstetrics, which remained in the hands of the midwives for over a thousand years. As a historian on childbirth across cultures, Brigitte Jordan notes: "Birth was then clearly considered women's business, a definition of the event that was shared, apparently, by all members of society. This view, it is worth noting, had religious and legal sanctions, as evidenced by the fate of a German physician who disguised himself as a woman in order to observe a birth. He was caught and burned at the stake in Hamburg in 1522."[11]

During and after the Renaissance, with the building of cities and hospitals, strangers began to attend to pregnant women.[12] The *accoucheur,* or male midwife, became popular after French king Louis XIV employed one for his favorite mistress.[13]

In the United States, male doctors began to supplant women in caring for pregnant women during the 18th century. Doctors started to provide advice, more like warnings, to pregnant women, including avoidance of the latest fashions that could threaten the health of the mother and the unborn baby.[14] By the 19th century, physicians and health reformers had displaced midwives and redefined pregnancy and childbirth as an illness, in part to create a market for their services.[15]

Many women, however, safeguarded their modesty or did not think male physicians could understand their symptoms. Others frowned on the idea of pregnancy as a disease that required a medical diagnosis.[16] However, geographic mobility made it more difficult for women to rely on their friends and family. Despite the turn to doctors, many women lived far from access to medical professionals. In fact, even in the early 20th century, *The Maternity Association,* an organization of nurses dedicated to providing medical support to pregnant women, sent nurses out into communities to find and offer advice. A 1930s guide for these nurses encourages that: "There are many ways of reaching them—talks to groups, newspaper articles, posted announcements in shop windows, stuffers in mail and packages; telling doctors, ministers, social workers, policemen, postmen, store-keepers, delivery men, and janitors about your service. But canvassing—the house to house, door to door search for the mothers—is the only sure way of finding every one and that only when some canvassing is a part of the every month's work."[17]

In time, most women assumed that doctors were the proper caregivers for pregnancy. With that, pregnancy shifted from a community affair to a medical experience.

Isolated Advice

A recent post in a pregnancy chat room queried, "I'm looking for some non-freak-my-shi**-out books about pregnancy."[18] The post went on to discuss a woman's dissatisfaction with the pregnancy advice books she found at her local bookstore. Several moms-to-be soon responded with suggestions of many different types of books for her. The ability for this woman to select a book that suits her tastes did not emerge overnight. An examination of the rise of pregnancy advice books can be understood within the context of the shifting of authority of pregnancy from religious to medical authorities.

Often cited as the first pregnancy advice book, *The Byrth of Mankynde, otherwyse named the Womans Booke* was published by Thomas Raynalde in 1540. A translation of an earlier German text,[19] the book's intended audience was women, but some worried that men might read the book for lewd purposes.[20] Writing about pregnancy during this time period was considered a politically charged act, in part because pregnancy and its depictions often were restricted by religious authority.[21]

Early advice books for pregnant women typically fall into one of two tracts: those written by medical professionals and those written by religious leaders. The medical texts, prior to the 19th century, most often were written to be read only by other medical professionals. For example, a midwife published in Europe in 1671 a book titled *The Midwives Book or the Whole Art of Midwifery Discovered: Directing Childbearing Women How to Behave Themselves,* instructing women about the medical issues of pregnancy. For example, the book suggests that pregnant women should "drink every morning a good draught of Sage Ale" in order to strengthen the womb.[22] The book also offers caution as to when something may be wrong: "The Child moves not though you wet your hand in warm water and rub it over her belly which is a true trial, and it will stir if it be alive."[23]

As women in the United States began to increasingly rely on the medical profession during pregnancy, they looked to outside experts for advice. This coincided with the growth of the publishing industry in the United States, which allowed for cheaper printing and a greater volume of books. In 1851, Congress authorized the United States Postal Office to deliver books with discounted rates, allowing people in small towns and rural areas to have access to information.[24] The rising rate of literacy coupled with the increasing availability of books influenced women's use of material that advised how to have and raise children. In the 18th and beginning of the 19th centuries, businesses discovered motherhood as an untapped market.[25] Consumer advice and information became available in books and magazines. Julia Grant and Ann Hulbert have both explored the rise and popularity of "baby experts" in the 19th century.[26] The rise of advice manuals for new mothers, particularly in the urban north in the 1800s, was a chance for these experts to influence mothers.[27]

While advice books for women grew in popularity during this period, they focused more on raising children rather than giving birth to them. Those that do focus on pregnancy are intended only for a medical audience, such as W. E. Fothergill's *Manual of Midwifery: For the Use of Students and Practitioners,* which discusses techniques for diagnosing pregnancy and treating women in labor.[28] Books that appealed directly to women approached pregnancy from a religious perspective, such as Reverend Thomas Searle's *A Companion for the Season of Maternal Solicitude,* which expressed the need to impart Christian values to the home of the pregnant woman.[29]

Eventually, during the 20th century, pregnancy advice books directed at women began to shed their religious nature and focused on advice from medical professionals. One such book, published in 1904, encouraged pregnant women to engage in moderate physical activity: "Exercise is the greatest preserver of health and beauty. It must, however, be taken under proper conditions and in moderation. Fresh air should be its invariable adjunct."[30] This author also brought up a topic that women might have been reluctant to mention to their doctor. He refers to: "Irritation and itching of the external parts. This is a most troublesome affection, and may occur at any time, but more especially during the latter period of the pregnancy; and as it is a subject that a lady is too delicate and too sensitive to consult a medical man about, I think it well to lay down a few rules for her relief."[31] The author's frank discussion is made possible by the fact that women are able to read this advice in solitude. Women distanced from their close social networks may have felt uncomfortable bringing up personal subjects in the presence of strange, male doctors, but the private nature of reading allows them to receive professional advice without fear or guilt.

As women began to read these books, experts accelerated their use by asserting the superior nature of their advice. A nurse touted her book as a resource for women who could now rely on a source other than a friend for advice. The author dismissed advice a woman may receive from her friends: "Their counsel was a mass of superstitious rubbish and ignorant chatter; harmful, or at best, useless remedies and the death-dealing assurance that it was time enough to call a doctor when the baby started to come."[32] Contrary to the conventional wisdom of the 19th century, this nurse advises to treat pregnancy as a normal condition: "Continue with the work, amusements and exercise that you are used to and enjoy except of course such activities as the doctor may forbid. In general, try to forget that you are pregnant, so far as you can do this and still remember to take proper care of yourself."[33]

Yet other medical professionals, such as Dr. Nicholas J. Eastman in his book *Expectant Motherhood,* still referred to pregnancy as a period of "confinement" and advised women about its negative aspects. Pregnant women were warned to be careful of too much driving in a car because it could cause fatigue.[34] In discussing employment and pregnancy, Dr. Eastman writes, "Although employers nowadays are very liberal-minded about such matters, there are naturally certain positions which cannot be held after the pregnancy becomes apparent. If this is a factor, plans should be made to discontinue work before the end of the fifth month."[35] This quote recalls a time when pregnancy was something to hide and safeguard from others, as a personal, private experience. The dominant mass medium of the time, print, helped to reinforce this perspective, as women read these books in private.

Of course, other social forces contributed to the privacy of pregnancy. One later advice book argues that the downsizing of the American family led to fewer occasions for young women to interact with pregnant women: "No wonder young women often see pregnancy, not as the usual female routine, but as something quite individual and unusual."[36] The book attempts to compensate by discussing issues affecting pregnant women, from their personal feelings to working during pregnancy.

Although sometimes contradictory, the advice of this period generally focuses on teaching expectant mothers to conform to public standards of decency while retaining her health during pregnancy. Today, though, advice is returning to the domain of the mother. *Unlike the Elephant* serves as a precursor to the advice books of today because it details pregnancy from the point of view of a pregnant woman, making it a rare advice book for its time. Sylvia Smeal, a woman in 1950s London, provides a personal account of her difficulty becoming pregnant and carrying her baby to term. She also describes in detail personal issues, like her morning sickness and heartburn,[37] and explores how being pregnant encourages others to share their personal pregnant experiences: "Until I began this pregnancy, I had found most of my friends and acquaintances reasonably restrained about their obstetric experiences. Now, they come out with the most extraordinary stories—and I repeat, extraordinary."[38]

Pregnancy during earlier periods was an unmediated experience, in the sense that women consulted other women to solicit advice for themselves. As social networks dissolved, they were replaced by a mediated experience in the form of published books. Initially, these books were written by those considered experts in the field, but they were experts who were excluded from the pregnant experience, as doctors and clergy were largely male callings. Smeal's book demonstrates the rebuilding of the social network of women, using the mediated form of the book, to provide women with advice from their peers.

The growth of advice books reflects an important shift in the networking of women. No longer is advice connected to a physical place or to whom one knows. Women can now receive messages in private, which echoes the biases of the printed word. Reading, by its nature, encourages a solitary experience. As women read these books and internalize their messages, the books and authors who write them become authorities. Yet, the authority of the book emerges simply from the fact that it is written and then published, which reifies its message as important and trustworthy. The act of printing changes a message by changing how people receive it. Hearing advice from family and friends is a communal experience focused on preserved wisdom. Reading in solitude advice written by "experts" objectifies the message and suppresses the reader as an active agent within her community. Removing the communal character of advice eradicates barriers against consumerism. Advice publishing is a business, and its books reflect the biases of the sender, whether they be the push for the medicalization of pregnancy, preconceptions about feminism, or ideals of what it means to be a good mother.

Specialized Advice

Today, pregnancy advice books can be found virtually everywhere. They have moved beyond the boundary of the bookstore to prominent displays in drugstores, department stores, and other retailers. A quick search on Amazon.com for "pregnancy advice books" yields over 400 results. These books also have expanded their market beyond pregnant women. An entire group of books are devoted to the pregnant dad, such as *The New Dad's Survival Guide*,[39] *The Father's Almanac*,[40] and *My Boys Can Swim!*[41] Publishers have categorized other books to pursue subsets of pregnant women. Some books target the pregnant teen, such as *The Unplanned Pregnancy Book for Teens and College Students.*[42] Just as many books have a medical focus, like Denise Austin's *Ultimate Pregnancy Book.*[43] This brings us to another category of advice books: advice from the celebrity. The two most popular titles in recent years are Brooke Shield's *Down Came the Rain: My Journey through Postpartum Depression,*[44] and Jenny McCarthy's *Belly Laughs.*[45]

The scale of publishing and marketing of these advice books is only one remarkable change in this industry; another is the frank discussion and specific language not evident in earlier books. For example, first-person accounts of pregnancy in the 1950s express its discomforts in only the vaguest sense. Compare this with just the titles of some of the chapters in McCarthy's book: Granny Panties (Letting Go of the G-String), Niagara in My Pants (Vaginal Discharge), and That Ain't My Ass! (Cellulite Gain). These, in fact, are some of the tamer chapters.

These books demonstrate that pregnancy has become a public experience, and its symptoms can be discussed with a new level of humor and openness. In the past, pregnancy advice books were useful to only pregnant women and their caretakers. Now, many of these books are marketed to and bought by fans wanting a glimpse into the inner lives of these stars. In fact, several book reviewers on Amazon.com have written that, after buying McCarthy's book for someone else who was pregnant, they read it though they were not pregnant themselves. Pregnant stars hawking their advice books are not confined to appearing only in parenting magazines; their pitches are made on nation-wide television programs and general-interest magazines watched and read by all women, pregnant or not, and quite a few men.

One of the most popular pregnancy advice books today is Vicki Iovine's *The Girlfriends' Guide to Pregnancy.*[46] This book is advertised as advice by regular moms for all pregnant women, and it illustrates the retrieval of communal advice sharing. At first, pregnancy books were written by "experts" who claim their role as authority figures. Thus, late 19th and early 20th century books are written both by doctors and nurses who gain their expert authority from their knowledge of the body and by ministers who claim their moral authority from a perceived higher authority. Now, advice books are written by celebrities and everyday moms who claim a knowledge that comes simply from experience. Iovine identifies her book as a return to the resources of the past: "When a woman found out she was pregnant, she naturally turned to the other women of her tribe. . .her mother, sisters, aunts, and friends."[47] Her book allows women who have experienced pregnancy to be the advice givers. In fact, the subtitle of her book reads "Everything Your Doctor Won't Tell You," which pits the book in opposition to older, established tomes by experts.

It is important to note, however, that the past recalled by Iovine embodied an environment where pregnant women were physically and socially connected to their advice givers. Although other women who have experienced pregnancy may have more insight than doctors, they are merely a new group of strangers giving advice to readers. At first, advice books supplanted communal advice systems with guidance from strangers who possessed some designated expertise; now, the advice givers are both strangers to the pregnant reader and have no professional credentials certifying the reliability of their knowledge. The growth of the Internet enables yet another shift to an environment where groups of virtual friends and strangers give advice to one another.

Virtual Communities

Many places have emerged online for pregnant women to visit and share their experiences with each other. Like other websites, pregnancy sites have embraced interactivity to attract and hold members. Among others, Ivillage.com has set up user-generated discussion areas, and Babycenter. com has both discussion forums arranged by topic and a birth club, where women can join lists based on their due date. I spent one year visiting Babycenter's discussion forums. Since I was pregnant myself at the time, I felt comfortable in their world. Although I did not participate but simply lurked, I came to look forward to their daily chats, sharing, questions, and problem solving. After getting to know these women through their words, I interviewed some of the forums' regular visitors about how they used this virtual world during their pregnancies.

Immersing one's self in the discussion forums, it becomes quickly apparent that they offer a space for pregnant woman to form virtual communities. In fact, had I not been pregnant myself at the time, I would have felt quite uncomfortable invading the forums, as the women there are protective of their community and verify that participants have a legitimate reason to be there. I quickly came to know these women, if only by their pseudonyms, and looked forward to hearing how their pregnancies and lives were progressing.

These forums encourage visitors to get to know one another. Babycenter requires each person to assume an identity that is posted for all to see. Each birth club is controlled by a moderator, who works to stimulate conversation and follow-ups to questions from other women. Many women have set routines when they visit. Some check the forums early each morning, often recognizing and addressing each other according to their handle or nickname. Participants use endearing greetings for each other, share pictures and baby name suggestions, and discuss husbands, their other children, and their hopes and dreams. Interestingly, on one day, some women were discussing how much they dislike receiving unsolicited advice from strangers.[48] Clearly, these postings show that they do not see each other as strangers, but as a type of friend. They appreciate the control that these forums allow them: they can choose when to solicit advice and when to ignore it, for there is no one to hold them accountable in real life.

A common theme that emerges from interviewing these women is the feeling of community and common experiences regarding their pregnancies and adjusting to motherhood. One woman, Abby, says, "It is great to talk to someone that is going through the same thing as me."[49] Frances, going through her second pregnancy, confides that it is "reassuring that, while everyone doesn't experience the exact same things, what I'm going through is still normal and there are others who understand."[50] Comparing advice she receives from books on pregnancy, she finds the forums "more realistic, not as black and white—so many different opinions."

Unlike the medium of print, the Internet is a technology that is non-hierarchical: no formal power structures control the creation and flow of information in the same way as mass media. One can see the significance of this characteristic within these forums. Unlike advice books, all participants can give advice to anyone else. And, though official moderators are assigned to these forums, no one responds more seriously to the advice from them than from others.

Also, unlike a book, because women can conduct an interactive conversation, the forums encourage them to see the advice and problems related to pregnancy as not absolute but in flux. This aspect of the technology allows women to have a relationship reminiscent of the companionship women received in earlier periods. For them, as well as these women, pregnancy was both a communal and individual experience, and women were able to talk about their pregnancies with other women as they experienced them. However, these earlier communities of women were not otherwise strangers; they were connected by location and need. Now, the Internet establishes connections using only the shared interest of pregnancy. In fact, through options available to them while signing in, women are allowed and even encouraged to remain anonymous and preserve their privacy, an option not offered to women in earlier times.

Some women choose to hide completely behind their handle and avatar, while others choose handles that reveal part or all of their identity. It is this feeling of anonymity that Abby says allows her to express her true feelings about aspects of her pregnancy: "I feel that when I share my experience with these women I am not being judged as I might be when I tell someone who has not been pregnant before. It is understood that I may be complaining and whining about my pregnancy but I am not unhappy being pregnant, I am more tired of the difficulty instead. This makes me feel like I am not alone and that there are many woman out there who understand."[51]

The lack of face-to-face communication allows women in these forums to express concerns or thoughts that they may repress in real life. Beth describes her time online as a freeing experience: "I am more comfortable there—I feel I can be myself."[52] Another woman confessed her disappointment when she found out she was having a second son, but she was not comfortable voicing that feeling publicly to people that she knew. Online, she found the support of other women who acknowledged her feelings.

Many women discussed their freedom to post embarrassing questions. Abby said, "I think it's easy to post certain things that would normally embarrass me because the people on the other end don't know who I am." An example of these questions comes from someone who posted online and asked:

I wanted to know if anyone else was having some dry "crusting" on or between the skin of your nipples (sorry to be so graphic). I've been curious today and found yellowish crust on both my nipples—Could it be dried up discharge? as my body "prepares for breastfeeding?" I'm 19.5 weeks and due August 9th . . . I'm excited with pregnant-fever but down with a terrible cough & cold . . . hope all is well with your belly.

Another woman responded and reassured her that this condition is perfectly normal. Another woman replied, "I'm glad I'm not the only one. I was really starting to wonder about it, I started noticing it a few weeks ago."[53] Another woman questioned:

Hopefully I don't sound too dumb with this one, but does anyone else have extremely itchy breasts? I don't remember this happening with any of my other pregnancies, but this time, they are so itchy all the time, I almost can't stand it!! lol I have started lotioning them up after my shower, and it has helped a tiny bit. But I feel like a freak, having to go into the bathroom to scratch them!![54]

Other women immediately replied to reassure her, offer her advice, and express their gratitude that they are not suffering from the same condition. These bulletin boards offer a chance for women to safely share publicly sometimes very private experiences.

Although the women repeatedly claim that they feel freer to talk and reveal within the bulletin board, a closer examination of the content of these bulletin boards shows the challenges these women face in defining and limiting their community. One woman cites an example of a posting that bothered her when someone responded to another woman's question about ultrasound. This woman was angry because the woman who responded was not pregnant.[55] Although the woman I interviewed was upset about the tone of these responses, it is clear that there were many who felt that unless you were pregnant, you had no place being in these forums. The pregnant community of the past is clearly different than the one here. Part of the definition of a community rests on the privilege the group has of choosing its members. Here, there is no way to know how many of the women visiting these bulletin boards are actually pregnant. In the past, men could be killed for trying to sneak a peek at a birth. Here, the community tries to be as tightly knit and defined, but that is impossible due to the constraints of the technology.

Occasionally, these posters extend their friendships beyond the forums, and they share more than their experiences as pregnant women. For example, Abby has met a friend that she now e-mails regularly. She thinks they will remain "friends," although she frames the word in quotes, acknowledging that this friend is different from her real-life ones.[56] Beth has met another poster who lives close by, and they have since become friends. In fact, she declared that this friend will serve as her backup to watch her first-born child when she goes in labor with her second.

Challenging the Medical Establishment

An examination of these virtual communities reveals that women have a new space in which to challenge formal, professional advice regarding their pregnancies. In the 19th century, women began to rely more on experts for information on child care. Although the information was not always scientific, it provided practical knowledge to help women make decisions and created a model for how a mother should act.[57] Now, these forums have become a place that allows women to treat each other as experts, oftentimes bypassing the traditional authority of medical professionals. Commonly, a woman poses a question about her doctor's recommendation that she disagrees with or has concerns about. Other women then frequently respond by acknowledging that she should listen to her doctor but qualify the recommendation with advice from their own experiences that differs from doctors or advice books. For example, one woman asks: "I just found out my in-laws want to throw me a shower in Tennessee and I live in Texas. My OB says no travel after 5/10/04 but I can't fit anymore travel into my schedule until at least mid-May or late May. Do you think it's okay to travel a few weeks past that date. I don't have any complications so far. Any advice or should I just call my OB?"[58]

The women I interviewed said that they sometimes save a call to the doctor by first consulting the forums. For instance, one woman asks whether she can receive an X-ray at the dentist. Several women quickly answer her with a definitive no.[59] Beth said that one of the reasons she went online in the first place was because she was having a difficult pregnancy: "I wanted answers to my questions that I didn't want to wait till my next appointment for."

Although online forums cannot serve in place of physical examinations, they allow women to give comfort and reassurance, roles once performed by doctors and nurses who now are increasingly under pressure from the efficiencies of the healthcare industry. When a woman posted her concern about not feeling enough movement, other mothers wrote in to tell her not to worry.[60] The woman went for her doctor's appointment and was told that her pregnancy was normal. Afterward, the other women asked with genuine concern about her doctor's assessment. For these women, the forums are a way of extending their medical care beyond visits to the doctor.

An examination of these forums suggests that, the weaker a woman's relationship was with her doctor, the more likely she would be to solicit the advice of the online community. Carol told me, "With my 1st pg I felt my dr. blew me off a lot, if I would have checked out the web I would have found that I wasn't the only one going through those things." Abby said she felt reassured about the multiple contractions she was feeling by other mothers who told her that this is common in second pregnancies. Frances, however, acknowledges that she values her midwife more that the forums because the midwife was more familiar with her personal history. Obtaining medical information from an alternate source, such as a trusted online community, becomes more appealing to women as the medical profession reduces doctors' face time with patients, in effect making them strangers.

In addition to medical advice, the forums allow women to discuss personal and social issues of pregnancy that would never be raised in the doctor's office. Abby said:

As far as relationships and family advice, I feel the bulletin board advice has been more helpful, I am able to communicate with others who have been in the same situations that I am in and find out how they dealt with the issues. Doctors don't have a lot of time in their offices to sit down and really talk about personal issues that are going on in your life besides the medical aspect. In chat rooms you have all the time to discuss and dissect the problem and find the answer or solution that is right for you.

With her medical issues, however, Abby goes straight to her doctor.[61] Marnie says that the advice has been helpful "because I don't have any friends with kids. So I've definitely been paying a lot of attention. Mostly lurking. I think Babycenter had a lot of good advice. I had no idea about how I should feel and what's normal." For these women, pregnancy is not merely a medical condition; it is social, too. They use these forums to learn how to deal with social aspects of their pregnancy or their impending changing lifestyle, much as women did before they fell under the care of medical professionals.

In fact, some feminists critique the medical profession for making the pregnant experience unnecessarily medically constrained within a system of patriarchy. The obstetrics field also represents to some a capitalist society dominated by technology, with women in labor just another group subject to the rules of the medical industry.[62] One may argue that these forums empower women to reshape how pregnancy can be defined and understood.

Although these online communities resemble the informal advice networks of women in the past, several important differences have created a distinct experience for pregnant women. In the past, a pregnancy was shared with women within a family or village who were physically present. Today, discussion forums and chat rooms have become an electronic village, where women can share their experiences with communities of their own choosing.

For many women, an online community can be freer and less judgmental than their real-life one. Pregnancy forums allow women to reveal personal concerns or private issues that they could not in real life. Doctors and other medical professionals began to take control over the pregnant experience in the 19th century; in the 21st century, women reclaimed control through the use of virtual communities, where they could have a newfound access to other women going through similar experiences. The asynchronous nature of the environment allows the women to ask and receive advice on their own time. However, virtual friends cannot serve the same function as a networked physical community. Pregnant women have regained informal networks of advice, but they have not recovered the physical network of women that supports them and identifies their pregnancy holistically within their everyday lives.

Public Pregnancies

Pregnancy discussion forums and chat rooms are virtual communities where women can choose whether and when to contribute; blogs are a way for women to publicly announce and update their pregnancies online. If the former is reminiscent of a community of women sharing advice, blogs are more akin to letter writing, with the addition of immediate feedback and the knowledge that the letter is public.

The openness of pregnancy blogs can be surprising. Before they start to show, women often post their ultrasounds to share, and some put up pictures of their pregnancy test showing a positive result. Many women post pictures of their bodies during their pregnancies. Bare tummies are common, with the bra and belly shot an artful variation.

One pregnant blogger I interviewed, Jodi, discussed what she chose to reveal and conceal: "There's very little that I didn't reveal—I talked about my breasts growing, hurting, and leaking. I talked about the aches and pains. I talked about the joys. I shared my ultrasounds and sound bites of the fetus's heartbeat. I talked about having gas (sheesh, looking back, I talked a LOT about having gas!). I talked about my cervix dilating and effacing." Yet, Jodi chose not to share the topless belly shots she took of herself. She only mailed them to select friends "mostly because I didn't want some pregnancy-fetishist to think of them as porn."

The open nature of blogging can be tempered by the perceived reception of content, which illustrates how the medium erodes boundaries between public and personal roles. Another blogger, Jeanne, described her husband's eagerness to share topless pictures of his pregnant wife when he created a pregnancy blog for her. She said, "His family was like whoa. I got to make the decision and I decided not to have them." Her decision was based in part by her concern that people with whom she had a professional relationship with could go online and see her nude.

The negotiation of what to share and keep private reveals how women struggle to separate the wholeness of their pregnancies within this media environment. Pregnancy affects a woman's whole body and is intimately physical. In the past, the seclusion of pregnant women constrained most of these physical changes to the private sphere. Online, each woman must choose which elements of her pregnancy she reveals publicly, and which parts she keeps private. Unlike virtual communities, where participants assume, or insist, that most readers are themselves pregnant, bloggers often recognize that anyone may visit a blog for any reason. Jodi, for instance, is conscious that she is writing for a public audience: "I know that many people hide their identities on their blog—I never had much thought to do that. . . . Each of my blog entries, on the other hand, is a 'piece'. I write them as little complete pieces, I go back and read and edit and try to make sure that they sound like I want them to. They're written to be shared, to be read, to be enjoyed."

Although bloggers often cite the desire to update friends and families about the pregnancy as the original purpose of creating a blog, readership usually extends past these people to strangers. Jodi set up a counter and discovered that over a hundred people had read her website. Instead of deterring her from sharing intimate details, this audience has encouraged her to write even more.

A YouTube clip proves that pregnancy can attract a large audience. A video of a man filming his pregnant wife's growing belly each day became one of the most-viewed videos on the website and rewarded the couple with a visit to the CBS's *The Early Show*.[63] The mother, Carlin, wrote on the couple's blog, "I mean, really, whoever thinks that their little home-movie project will be something that people really want to see, not just be subjected to when they're over for dinner?"[64]

Many blogs are filled with venting about uncontrollable cravings or some of the other side effects of pregnancy. In this way, blogs differ from chat rooms and discussion forums because they often simply reveal emotions rather than share advice. Another pregnant blogger, Jocelyn, reveals how blogs are used to compensate for the isolation of modern pregnancy: "I also think it has made me closer with some of my family members that I don't get to see as much as I'd like. This is one of the first babies of my generation on my mom's side, so everyone is really excited, but we're all very busy. This was just one way to keep everyone connected, with little effort on either side."

Although they are informed, these relatives are only virtually connected to the pregnancy. In the past, extended family served as a support network for a pregnant woman. Now, they are merely an audience to the online show. Although most bloggers do offer a section for visitors to write comments and give feedback, these areas are mostly a place for relatives and friends to cheer on the pregnancy rather than to advise or support the pregnant woman.

Jocelyn waited until her second trimester to begin her blog because she said it was important to her to hold off the public announcement of her pregnancy. Despite the changes this new media environment has brought, some traditions from the past, such as keeping a pregnancy hidden until the mother feels more secure about the status of the pregnancy, have carried over to the present. Like Jodi, Jocelyn is aware of her audience and writes with them in mind, not as she would in a private journal:

> I've tried to keep it rated "PG" since my family members and friends are reading it. I give them details, but I realize that they don't want all of the gory info. I've also tried to stay positive so that I don't regret some of the things I've written. You're pretty hormonal when you're pregnant, so it wasn't always easy—and I know my mood shifts certainly snuck in during some posts—but for the most part, I just tried to use it as more of a log of pregnancy highlights, both good and bad.

For both Jocelyn and Jodi, their blogs have become an important place to preserve the pregnancies for themselves and their babies. Jeanne describes her blog as her baby's virtual baby book. She has created an area where people can offer possible baby names and imagines that her future child will want to see what he or she could have been named. Thus, the pregnancy blog serves not only the present audiences of family, friends, and strangers, but also the future audience of the baby itself.

Conclusions: The Commoditization of Advice

The early history of pregnancy advice reveals a nonformal but vibrant social system in which friends, neighbors, and relatives shared in the pregnancy experience. Later, the professional medical establishment replaced this support network, and women were told to turn to doctors for pregnancy advice. As pregnancy moved from a socially defined experience to a medical one, the introduction of the pregnancy advice book became a boon for the publishing industry. Women began to actively seek out advice, rather than passively have advice brought to them. At the same time, women became increasingly isolated from interpersonal advice networks. Throughout these periods, thanks to both the social stigma of openly discussing pregnancy issues and the loss of a physically copresent advice network, pregnancy remained an intensely private experience for women.

Today, new media are changing again the information environment in which pregnant women receive advice and support, transforming pregnancy into a public experience. Discussion boards and chat rooms offer women new communities in which they can express their views, often without the harsh judgment that may be imposed on them by their real-life friends. Retrieving the earlier experience of communal information sharing, this new environment allows pregnancy to return to being as much a social experience as a medical one. Women now seek advice from both trained medical professionals and experienced women they find online.

The history of pregnancy advice has shifted from a social experience, to a medical one, to a combined social/medical one. Women tend to rely on doctors for some aspects of their pregnancy but now look to other communities, including virtual ones, to explore personal and social issues once discussed among networks of copresent women. As pregnant women became isolated from advice communities in the 19th century, consumerism filled the void. Advice once freely given by close family and friends was now offered by the marketplace, for a price.

Today, the pregnancy advice industry is stronger than ever. Celebrities routinely sell pregnancy advice books, and the bookselling giant Barnes & Noble recently entered the fray with its acquisition of the 700-page pregnancy reference book *Great Expectations*. Rather than restrict its marketing to pregnant women, the bookseller announced its venture with a full-page advertisement in the *New York Times*.[65] Discussion forums like Ivillage and Babycenter are sprouting up to provide places for pregnant women to congregate, but unlike past advice networks, these virtual communities must navigate around the advertising space that these websites sell. As pregnancy becomes commoditized, pregnancy advice purveyors seek out new audiences to expand their market. Once the pool of pregnant women who buy advice books, watch pregnant celebrity interviews on television, and view pregnancy blogs is exhausted, continued growth creates a public of pregnancy voyeurs, and pregnancy shifts from a private to public experience.

Chapter 4

A Pregnant Pause

Pregnancy and Popular Culture

In an episode of *All in the Family* where Gloria is pregnant and her husband Mike is showing Edith all the things they are doing to prepare for the delivery, Gloria's mother Edith, says "I'm glad I had Gloria when I did. I don't think I'd know enough to have a baby today."[1] Edith's comment illustrates the change in pregnancy as represented in popular culture in the past 50 years. It used to be that little was known or shown about pregnancy 50 years ago. As illustrated in the previous chapters, even the mother, particularly in the first part of the 20th century, did not always have much control over her pregnancy. She submitted to the control of the doctor and hospital and did what she was told. These days pregnant women and their husbands, as well as extended families, are all involved in the entire pregnancy process—from looking at a pregnancy test together, to being there for the first sonogram, and accompanying the mother in the delivery room. Television shows and films have also reflected this shift in the presentation of pregnancy by illustrating the changing role and involvement of the father, the exposing of the secrets of getting pregnant and infertility, by carefully depicting the sex involved in conception while still desexualizing the pregnant mother, and by reflecting the shifting anxieties of the public over pregnancy and the influence of technology on pregnancy. This chapter explores shifts in how pregnancy has been shown and covered in popular culture over time.

Conception: From Magic to Struggle

Stories about women trying to get pregnant are not necessarily abundant in early literature or very graphic, but they do exist. Probably the most celebrated examples are from biblical stories, including that of the famous Sarah, wife of Abraham, who does not become pregnant until well into her old age. In another biblical story, Hannah (wife of Elkanah) prays to God to grant her a child and then she is finally blessed with the arrival of Samuel. Debora Spar, author of *The Baby Business,* discusses how in biblical and ancient readings, infertility was typically blamed on the mother. She was required to resolve the problem on her own and Hannah praying to God for such a resolution is a good example.[2] A recent popular fiction book, *The Red Tent,* delves into the women characters of the bible and their relationship to each other, pregnancy, and motherhood.[3] While most people would immediately recognize the Brothers Grimm fairytale of *Rapunzel,* few realize the significance that pregnancy played in the original story. *Rapunzel* is about a couple who have great difficulty in conceiving a child. When the wife finally gets pregnant she develops a strong craving for a certain plant ("Rapunzel" or "Rampion" depending on the version). The wife or husband (depending on the version) keeps stealing this plant from the garden of a nearby enchantress or witch named "Dame Gothel" in order to feed her cravings because of their fear that the wife will die of her craving. Eventually the enchantress discovers the theft and confiscates the newborn child as payment and names her Rapunzel. When the child reaches maturity the enchantress locks her in a high tower without access from the outside. Eventually, the girl's long hair made into braids provides the means for a passing prince to gain access. In some versions of the story the child in the story ends up pregnant herself.[4] But, who remembers that version of the story? Instead, pregnancy, in early stories, was often minimized and hidden. But, since the mid-20th century, we have seen pregnancy introduced into early television and film.

Fans often say that one of their favorite episodes of *I Love Lucy* was the one where Ricky finds out that Lucy is pregnant. The entire episode rests on Lucy surprising Ricky with the news of her pregnancy. She can never find the right moment to tell him and finally has him perform a dance number "You're having my baby" at his club and surprising him with the news that he is actually singing for her.[5] This is a memorable episode not only for its poignancy but also because everyone is surprised by the news: Lucy, Ricky, and the fans. I also remember enjoying this episode but today the story strikes me as odd. These days, the husband is often as involved in the planning for the baby and knowledgeable of the woman's menstrual cycle as the woman herself. Today, men and women are in control of the fertility process and the hidden side of getting pregnant is exposed. Looking at the history of pregnancy representation on television illustrates television shifting to this new standard of fertility rituals in which the husband and wife play an equal part.

As in the *I love Lucy* episode, Gloria's first pregnancy in *All in the Family* comes as a surprise to both Gloria and her husband Mike. They are ambivalent because they were committed to not having children. However, she loses the baby by the end of the episode. When she gets pregnant again Gloria now tells her parents before her husband. When her mother Edith says she cannot believe that Mike does not know, her father Archie says "What business is it of his?"[6] While the line is meant to elicit a laugh, it also reveals a truth: fathers, in those days are just barely part of the process—needed only for conception and then later for fatherhood—but not during the pregnancy. In *Bewitched,* Samantha is not so much surprised but excited by the news of her pregnancy. She can't wait to surprise her husband with the news.[7] It is their first anniversary and Darrin is accidentally turned into a chimp, making it frustrating for Samantha to find the right moment to tell him the news. This episode illustrates the popular depiction of the father in pregnancy perfectly: he's just a "monkey" when it comes to pregnancy—clearly he had a part in the conception and will play the role of the father, but other than that, he's useless.

This idea of surprising the husband with the news continues on sitcoms. On *Full House* (a 1980s sitcom), Rebecca surprises Jessica by announcing that she is pregnant on the final episode of season 4. She arranges for all different little types of foods in an effort to convince him to guess that she's pregnant and when he does not, she does a charades type game with the family to announce the pregnancy to them. Jesse is also surprised and pleased.[8] Pregnancy is such a surprise that breaking the news of it becomes a part of the plot.

Today's surprise pregnancies are usually framed as an accident, an unplanned pregnancy, where the character may hesitate slightly before embracing it. On the second season finale of *Parenthood,* Kristina's third pregnancy is a surprise to both her and her husband. In the season finale of *Modern Family,* Gloria has a surprise pregnancy. On the season 6 finale of *Bones,* Dr. Brennan finds out she's pregnant. In these shows, the characters are surprised and ambivalent because they really did not expect this pregnancy. In the earlier shows of the 1960s, 1970s, and early 1980s, the characters often act surprised despite the fact that pregnancy in this stage in their life would not be unusual and might even have been planned. The viewers are left to assume that some type of birth control did not work out, though none of the shows actually discuss this. Preventing conception is sometimes mentioned in television programs today (the most famous example being an entire episode of Seinfeld revolving around Elaine's favorite sponge company going out of business), but it is infertility and the quest to get pregnant that is discussed much more often.

Infertility: The Quest for a Baby

In today's representation of the desire to get pregnant, television demonstrates how the outside forces of modern life interfere with conception, with biology getting in the way of a relationship, and the increase in knowledge of medical information creating new problems. As efforts to depict pregnancy increase, infertility or the struggle to become pregnant becomes a central component to the plot. Today, infertile women on television are a part of the plot or subplot of many television programs. In *Mad About You* (1992–1998), Jamie and Paul have difficulty conceiving, spanning season 4 of the program and leading to troubles in their marriage. At points they both undergo fertility testing and try alternative fertility methods. In *Friends*, Monica has trouble conceiving after talking about her desires to have a baby since the initial season of the program. In fact, she had even given up an earlier relationship because the man did not want children. When Monica and Chandler finally get married and try for children, they realize after many numerous efforts that they both have fertility problems. In one memorable episode, Monica has timed her ovulation cycle so that Chandler needs to have sex with her that evening but then they get in a fight and he refuses sex.[9] She then pretends to no longer be angry with him in order to resolve the fight just so that he can have sex with her. In this episode, not only do viewers get a window into fertility efforts but you also see the woman facing difficulty in trying to control her cycle while needing the involvement of her husband, who is also aware of the cycle. It is evident here that there is a conflict between biology and the relationship. The couple's fight and relationship need to take a backseat to their obligation or desire to get pregnant: sex needs to happen whether or not they are in the mood, a challenge that television shows us is experienced by all couples facing infertility. We see this as early as the 1980s, in an episode of *Thirtysomething*, where Michael and Hope are trying to conceive their second child and need to hire a babysitter so that they have time to have sex at the right moment in her cycle. The moment is not romantic, and Hope tells Michael "The earth doesn't have to move every time," but it is clear that both members of the couple miss their "real" sex life versus this timed sex based on the woman's cycle.[10] Television reflects the shift between the two—sex for pleasure versus sex for procreation.

In other plotlines, the reality of modern life interferes with conception. In *King of Queens,* Carrie and Doug are trying to get pregnant again (after a previous miscarriage) and have difficulties in finding the privacy that they need. In one episode, Doug has to hire someone to take Carrie's dad (who is living with them) out for walks, so that they have the time to try to conceive.[11] In another episode, Doug's parents visit, providing them with no privacy during her fertile window. In these scenes, Doug and Carrie are struggling with outside forces because while both of them are deeply committed to getting pregnant, they are not yet ready to reveal their desire to get pregnant to their extended family.[12] For Doug and Carrie, getting pregnant is still a private moment because otherwise it would be akin to announcing their sex life. Unlike in the 1950s and 1960s, where conception is hidden to the viewers, here, not only is it public, but both the man and the woman are in it together, both emotionally and physically. Pregnancy becomes even more public when Marshall and Lily share their progress in fertility efforts with their friends and family during the 2010–2011 fertility storyline of *How I Met Your Mother.* In one episode, Marshall tells his father that they are trying to conceive, prompting the father to become overly involved in offering advice, which Lily finds both bothersome and inappropriate. Lily and Marshall, disagreeing on whether they want a boy or girl, clash when they both secretly use various techniques to influence the sex of the baby.[13]

In *Notes from the Underbelly,* which involves following a pregnant couple throughout the pregnancy, crossing over different seasons, it is the husband who is more interested in having a baby than his wife and thus begins to read the books and take pleasure in taking control over the conception process.[14] The comedy from these programs arises from the conflict over whether the man or the woman is more vested in the process. But, the comedy for all these shows is also reflected in the fact that sex shifts from being private to public, sometimes against the desires of the couple.

Television dramas in the 21st century often represent infertility and the difficulties of getting pregnant in a more serious tone, reflecting the emotional struggles of the characters and also the cost that access to new and alternative medical technologies has on the couple. In *Brothers and Sisters,* an ABC show in its second season features one of the lead characters, Kitty, struggling with infertility, and the program shows her discussing her options with her doctor and having sex with her husband then sitting with her legs up in the air in an effort to increase her odds of getting pregnant. The couple visits doctors to discuss the different procedures and eventually think that adoption may be better suited for them. Kitty has a conversation with her sister where they discuss her sister's visit to Kitty's apartment during her last pregnancy and how the sister remembers the heartburn and Kitty remembers the baby kicking and feeling so alive. The sister reminds Kitty that the baby "remembers nothing." The sister is telling Kitty that the end result, the baby, is more important than the way she gets pregnant, although Kitty is more ambivalent about whether this is so. She grieves at her loss, and the struggle to become pregnant becomes a bone of contention between her and her husband. This is actually the second struggle with infertility the program has depicted. In the previous season, Kitty's sister-in-law could not get pregnant with her husband's sperm and asked his brother for a donation of his sperm. Discussion and disagreement ensued over which brother's sperm to use and they finally decided to have both brothers donate sperm and not have the doctor tell them which one is used. New medical techniques here are raising interesting questions about methods of conception as well as ethical and biological issues.

We also see changing notions of conception in stories that move beyond the traditional family. In one episode of *Modern Family*, gay couple Cam and Mitchell is out to dinner with Mitchell's sister Claire and her husband Phil.[15] When both couples drink a bit too much, Claire offers to donate her eggs so that Cam can contribute his sperm and they can "mix it and put in a surrogate lady thing." In the morning, though, everyone has second thoughts, and Cam and Mitchell decide to continue with their adoption plans.

Films also reflect how baby-making is changing. In the 2008 film *Baby Mama*, Kate (Tina Fey) hires Angie (Amy Poehler) to be a surrogate.[16] Kate alternatively pampers and controls Angie to protect the fetus, only to learn that the baby is not genetically hers, but belongs to Angie and her boyfriend. By the end of the film, Angie is raising her child, and Kate has become pregnant with her new boyfriend. In *The Back-Up Plan*, a movie released in 2010, Jennifer Lopez plays a woman who decides to use intra-uterine insemination to get pregnant after failing to meet the right man but still desires to have a baby.[17] Once pregnant, however, she finally meets her perfect man, but he is hesitant to get involved with her. He realizes by the end of the movie, though, that even if he did not help conceive this baby, he can still be a father to it. In *The Switch*, also released in 2010, Kassie (Jennifer Aniston) decides to buy sperm so she can start a family on her own. She even has a "conception party," where she invites all her friends over, and at the end of the party, she will impregnate herself with the sperm.[18] Chaos ensues, though, when her friend Wally (Jason Bateman) accidentally destroys the sperm and decides to substitute his own. These films all question the notion of parenthood, genetics, and what it means to be a family. Some of the films, such as *Baby Mama* and *The Switch*, reinforce the idea of the importance of genetic ties, while *The Back-Up Plan* promotes the idea that the family is defined by who decides to raise the child, though the end of this film brings back the traditional notion of genetic ties by showing that Kate has now become pregnant with her new boyfriend's baby as well.

In *Sex and the City*, the character of Charlotte was infertile and struggled through episodes trying to get pregnant and trying all different infertility remedies, including acupuncture. The struggle takes over her life and interferes with her first marriage. Other drama programs, like HBO's *Tell Me That You Love Me*, also feature the desire to become pregnant as a key component of the plot. The young married couple featured in this drama, are struggling to become pregnant and it affects their marriage. Since the show is on cable, it is bound by fewer restrictions regarding nudity and suggestive connotations and shows the couple having sex as well as the woman peeing on a stick, hoping that she is pregnant. The inability to get pregnant affects this couple's relationship deeply and the struggles they face are shown by the program.

In all these TV programs, there is a shift away from the idea of magical conception implied from the 1950s through the 1980s to the real challenges of getting pregnant. The trailer to the 2012 film, *What to Expect When You're Expecting* takes all the mystery out of conception saying "It's Too Late to Pull out Now." In the past, women were often surprised to find themselves pregnant, but now women are shown making great efforts to conceive and conception no longer seems magical but also no longer is it guaranteed. This representation reflects the biological challenges of women as they face the question of whether they should have babies while young to match their best biological chance of conception or whether should continue to work professionally and achieve other goals before shifting to becoming a mother. As women face these conflicting issues, television is reflecting these same challenges. Also reflected here is the changing involvement of men in the process. The man is no longer the chimp depicted on *Bewitched*. Now, men are both willing and involved participants in the conception process and the woman is no longer the sole proprietor of the knowledge of her cycle. In the *Friend*'s episode you see Chandler withholding his sperm in order to have control over Monica during their fight. In addition, when blame is attributed to the lack of ability to conceive, it is no longer the exclusive fault of the mother. In *Friends*, both characters have the problem. The challenge of keeping sex a private, marital pleasure for a couple while also trying to conceive becomes another problem for real-life couples as well as the ones depicted in popular culture. Fans of these programs have grown accustomed to watching their favorite characters conceive. One TV blog site encouraged others to root for which character will get pregnant first, *Grey's Anatomy*'s Meredith or *How I Met your Mother*'s Lily.[19]

Putting the Sex Back in Pregnancy

In *All in the Family,* when Gloria announced her pregnancy, her father Archie says, "Bad girls get pregnant. Nice married girls is always expecting." This joke is a commentary not only on how society considered pregnancy a word charged with meaning but also a nod to the episodes of *I Love Lucy,* which were not even allowed to utter the word "pregnant." Archie is also raising the idea that inevitably, the announcement of a pregnancy could not help but trigger an acknowledgement that a woman has had sex.[20] In a similar moment, in the film *Father of the Bride Part II* (1995), with Steve Martin (a remake, in fact), the father is very pleased with his son-in-law until he finds out that his daughter's pregnant (news that seems to be a surprise only to him). Then he suddenly becomes suspicious of his son-in-law for "doing this" to his daughter. Pregnant women in media have generally conformed to the biblical standard of the Virgin Mary, pregnant, beautiful, and with child but still a virgin in a sense that sexual beings and even the act of sex, which is of course, centrally connected to the notion of pregnancy, is absent from the idea of a pregnant woman. At first television programs hardly ever discussed sex and pregnancy, but today, the act of having sex to get pregnant has become an integral part of the plot of many programs. But television has been careful also to differentiate the act of sex so that there is "fun sex" and there is "conception sex," and both are represented on television in different ways.

Although television has long broken the barrier of displaying sex on the air, the characters still struggle with the idea of conception sex as a private subject. This is seen in the show *King of Queens,* when Doug and Carrie have trouble conceiving because of the presence of their in-laws. In *Brothers and Sisters* ("For the Children"), when Julia and Thomas are trying to get pregnant, they adopt an awkward sexual position. The viewer quickly learns that the wife learned about this position from her "TTC friends." This means her "trying to conceive" chat room and her husband is only partially joking when he asks, "And this is what you talk about in your chat rooms? With Strangers?"[21] In truth, he is annoyed with her discussion of their private sex life in a public setting. In these instances, the couple is wrestling with the fact that sex is generally considered a private act between the couple, but when having difficulty conceiving, it sometimes becomes necessary to let outsiders in on their private struggles.

Television though, has sex and sexual situations on television all the time. Most sitcoms have at least two characters who are working through some type of attraction for one another. Sex for pleasure occupies the time of lots of other characters or even complete programs, like HBOs *Sex and the City* or *Entourage.* The idea that sex sells is a popular adage for advertising on television. In truth, many advertisements on television are for some type of product that will make a person more sexually desirable, whether this is a hair product, skin cream, perfume, weight loss program, or food. For other products, like beer or soda, sex is often used to sell viewers by promising them a fun lifestyle filled with members (usually of the opposite sex) who will find them attractive and fun to be around.

Sex then is a popular and driving economic force behind television. But, when it comes to conception sex, television must be careful in its presentation. Conception sex is sex for its purest purpose—giving life. One might think that even religious figures would not object to a discussion of conception sex but for television, it poses a problem. Conception sex means that sex isn't fun and useful for advertising or selling anymore because it connects sex with its ultimate purpose, which is bringing life into the world. This certainly does not put people in the mood to do what television needs them to do: buy. Television solves this problem by differentiating everyday sex as "fun sex" and conception sex as "work sex." Most scenes that feature couples trying to have a baby do not involve couples enjoying themselves or in the throes of passion. Instead, it is about couples having to work hard at it, interfering with their marriage, their jobs, and their enjoyment of life. The fun act of sex is subsumed by attempts to conceive, and sex becomes part of a struggle within the couple, a battle between the couple and biology, and the need to use medical science to battle biology.

Once a woman is pregnant, she is allowed to retain her sexuality but within limits. If she demands too much sex from her husband, she is portrayed in a comic way, with the program feeling sorry for the husband. In films, pregnant women have been seen having sex, but typically the awkwardness of the pregnancy is part of what leads to the comic moments. In the film *Nine Months,* the male lead played by Hugh Grant is not happy about becoming a father in the first place. When his girlfriend starts becoming interested sexually, he images her as a giant insect and he is her prey.[22] In the film *Knocked Up,* the characters are trying to have sex though she is visibly pregnant.[23] She wants him to "go deeper" but he's worried that he'll hurt the baby, and they actually fight about it while having sex.

It's a funny moment for the film, showcasing the pregnant woman as having a stronger sex drive than her boyfriend.

Yet, this could be changing as there are now a few films where pregnant women engage in passionate moments where the sex is not functioning as comic relief, such as a scene in the film *Munich,* where the wife and husband embrace passionately after he returns from being away.[24] In the film *Waitress,* the character is a pregnant woman who begins an affair with her obstetrician.[25] Although her sexuality is a central part of the film, she is somewhat detached from her pregnancy, and the film thus reflects her ambivalent feelings about her sexuality and her ability to be a strong mother. Here, pregnancy is no longer a debilitating condition, and sex after conception is still considered fun.

In reality TV programs, in particular, sex is starting to become a welcome subject for discussion. Tori and Dean's *Inn Love* was the first American reality program where the pregnant woman, Tori Spelling, was the star. The premise of the program is that Spelling, a former child actress and daughter of the famous television producer Aaron Spelling, decided with her husband, Dean (also an actor), to open up an inn. A key feature of the program is that Tori is well into her pregnancy when they undertake this project. In this program, sex is exposed rather than hidden as Tori and Dean appear to have an active sex life despite her pregnancy. However, we do at times see her concerns for the baby. For example, in one episode, she goes to the doctor because she is worried that their rough sex may have hurt the baby. The doctor has to reassure her that the baby is okay. In the third season of the program, Tori is pregnant again and though we don't see them in romantic, sexual situations as often, Tori is consumed about not being sexy, and whether her husband will end up attracted to his scuba teacher rather than her. But it is obvious that they still value their sex life, where in one episode when Tori is about to leave on a trip, Dean asks her if she has time for some "pre-flight sex."[26]

Another program that follows a pregnancy is *Scott Baio is 46 . . . and Pregnant.* Scott Baio, yet another former child star, has just found out his future wife is pregnant and the show features his adjustment (or lack thereof) to his impending parenthood. But Scott is not afraid to express his sexual desires for his pregnant wife. Scott makes it clear that he is in the mood for more sex with his pregnant wife and a prenatal yoga type class has put him in the mood. He even comments that the sounds of her giving birth remind him of sex. In fact the natural childbirth approaches to labor and delivery encourages women to tap into their sexual side. There is a connection between sex and the entire pregnancy process. Although the program represents Scott as a bit over-the-top in his sexualized feelings, in fact, his feelings are a natural part of pregnancy. Thus, these two programs are the closest programs on television to actually connecting sex and pregnancy.[27]

Allowing sex to become a part of the representation of pregnancy allows for a more realistic depiction of pregnancy. However, in the program *A Baby Story,* where of course it is obvious that the couple must have had sex to get pregnant, sex is not discussed by them. *A Baby Story,* which is on the Learning Channel, part of the Discovery Network, follows a couple through the birth of their child. Each program is set up so that they begin following the mother shortly before she is ready to give birth until the eventual birth of the baby. Sex is ignored in favor of the focus being simply on the fears and excitement the couple has for their forthcoming child. Sure, sex is needed to get pregnant, but once pregnant, the woman needs to stay focused on her expanding belly and maternal desires: the pregnant woman is desexualized.

Although the subject of sex is increasingly discussed and visible on television, it needs to be sex for pleasure rather than sex for conception, which is relegated to something couples do as work because they have to. Once pregnant, the women are allowed to retain some degree of sexuality, depending on the program. Celebrity reality programs are more willing to uncover the sexy pregnant woman, while the typical documentary style baby program retains the mother in her Virgin Mary image. Sex may sell, but pregnant sex has its limits the programs seem to say.

Early Bonding: The Pregnancy Test and the Sonogram

In the past when a woman was found to be pregnant on television, the episodes mostly revolved around the comedy that the physical aspect the pregnant woman presented, with her expanding belly and the clumsiness and the decline in her physical agility. But, now it has become easier to visually represent pregnancy with two key inventions discussed more fully in a previous chapter (the pregnancy test and the sonogram). It is no surprise that writers and producers would begin to incorporate these developments as moments into their programs and films not only to give the viewers a similar experience that pregnant women actually face but also, because these visual moments, allow the viewers to attach to the pregnancy earlier in the process. On early television shows, the women had to have a phone call from her doctor in order to confirm her pregnancy and then she would share the news with the rest of her family. But now, the test allows a couple to find out together that they are pregnant, for friends or relatives to find out about the pregnancy from a pregnancy test "accidentally" left to be discovered, or sometimes it allows for a private moment between the audience and the pregnant woman alone as she finds out. In *Notes from the Underbelly,* the couple is able to share the moment together. In *Tell me that You Love Me,* the couple is haunted by the pregnancy test as it is so often negative. In *Friends,* Monica discovers the pregnancy test and Phoebe takes the credit for it—creating a comic episode for the gang. In *Beverly Hills 90210,* the parents find out that Brenda took a pregnancy test when they find her test in the garbage.[28] In the latest program representing teen pregnancy, the young girl hides her pregnancy test in her musical instrument and then privately takes the test, which comes out positive.[29] In the film *Knocked Up,* the revealing pregnancy test moment is shared by the sister and the lead character as again, tons of tests are bought so she can be absolutely sure. And, the sister even takes a test to compare results. The pregnancy test, then, moves from being controlled by the medical profession to being shared by the woman herself and whoever she chooses to include in the process. This allows for increased discussion about whether a woman wants the pregnancy. Further, it allows more people to become aware of the pregnancy earlier in the process. This mirrors real life as more people become a part of the pregnancy experience earlier in the process. The test also allows time for more controversy in the TV or movie program because you can test earlier. In the past, by the time the woman got to the doctor, she was probably pretty aware that there was a high likelihood of being pregnant. With the modern pregnancy test, you can test earlier in the process thus allowing a big moment of revelation to become the showcase of the show.

The sonogram episode also has begun to take up a central role in popular depictions of pregnancy, particularly in film and television, where it has become a type of pre-birth experience. Prior to widespread use of ultrasound, the birth of the baby or when it made its physical entrance, was the key moment in the film or the television episode. But now sonogram technology allows real-life parents as well as fictional ones, to meet their baby earlier. In television, the image is everything, while in real life, the birth is more real than an image of the baby shown on a sonogram. But on television the sonogram and the birth are both images; so in many ways they are equivalent in strength. The viewers are never going to get further than the screen in getting to meet this baby. This is seen in an episode of the program *Live with Regis & Kelly.* In a demonstration of the new 3-D ultrasound, Kelly Ripa, the cohost of *Live with Regis & Kelly,* viewed her baby live on an ultrasound. She became emotional during this moment, serving to bond the audiences to her and her pregnancy. She and the baby-to-be were humanized for the audience. Women could watch Kelly as just another pregnant mom going through the routine experience of a sonogram (although most women have yet to have the opportunity to experience a 3-D ultrasound). Likewise, in several episodes of *A Baby Story*, the sonogram moment appears frequently and thus allows viewers to not only see the image of the unborn child but also reassures them that the husband and wife have bonded to the baby by the use of the ultrasound. The ultrasound experience thus allows the audience to bond with the baby-to-be. Of course the audience bonds to an image rather than the baby but to the audience they are one in the same because they will never experience the real thing. Sometimes, though, an alternate view of the ultrasound moment is offered. Tina Fey, appearing on *Conan,* jokes with O'Brien that her 3-D sonogram image is a bit upsetting. She then displays an image that seemingly shows a monster-like fetus growing inside her. The joke plays on the disconnect between sometimes-creepy sonograms and the social expectation that people react with reverence and sentiment.[30]

Both in television and film, the ultrasound moment has been used as a way for the story to bring the father into the pregnancy. In fact this is true even in cases where the mother and father are no longer together. For example, in *Friends* there were actually two pregnancies that involved the character of Ross.[31] In the first, Ross's lesbian ex-wife is expecting. In the second, his on-again, off-again love Rachel is pregnant although they are no longer a couple. Both sonogram experiences give the father a chance to bond with the mother of his child. In the first pregnancy, Ross is fighting with his ex-wife and her new lover until he hears the sound of his baby's heart beating and sees his child for the first time.[32] The ultrasound experience allows Ross to transcend all else in order to bond with his child. Ross goes with Rachel for her ultrasound and ends up actually identifying the fetus to Rachel who cannot seem to see her baby in the sonogram. Ross uses the ultrasound experience to show that he is not only a father but also a father who can "find" his child. Ross's ability to transcend ultrasound technology by interpreting it for Rachel, allows him to still retain his masculinity while still becoming involved in the pregnancy.[33] The ultrasound is a safe way for the men to pierce the shield of control that the women have over the pregnancies. This is also seen in the program *7th Heaven,* when the ultrasound experience is used by Eric to cheer Annie up who is having some pregnancy blues. After failing miserably at every effort he makes to support Annie through her pregnancy, he arranges a special ultrasound for their anniversary and together they find out that they are having twins. Before the ultrasound, Eric was portrayed as a bumbling father who just cannot understand his pregnant wife.[34] But the ultrasound allows him to regain control and to become and feel useful. Television and film also reflects the ultrasound as a moment where the fathers are able to bond with the pregnancy in a way that could not happen before. In the television sitcom (airing 1987–1995), the character of Jesse, finds out through a sonogram that he is going to father twins and then the rest of the episode deals with his fears of fatherhood. In the film, *Nine Months*,[35] Hugh Grant's character is disconnected from his girlfriend's pregnancy. It is not until the ultrasound (which he misses by showing up late) that he realizes that he should become more involved. The doctor gives him a copy of the video of the ultrasound that he watches and which transforms him into a father. This is also seen in the TV show *Felicity* during the *Paper Chase* episode when Ben shows off the sonogram of his unborn child (with a woman with whom he had a one night stand) to his friend Sean who teases him for bonding with his future child. Similarly in the film *Knocked Up*, the father-to-be (after yet another one night stand) is in the role of providing comfort to the mother-to-be after the sonogram makes the experience all too real to her (she bursts into hysterics).

The ultrasound moment is critical to depictions of pregnancy in modern TV shows and films and is the source of much humor and comedy. For example, in the film *Juno*, the unmarried and pregnant teenager appears for an ultrasound along with her friend and stepmother.[36] The teenager is rather harshly judged by the ultrasound technician who is then yelled at by Juno's stepmother. The technician crosses a line in expressing her opinion because a technician is generally expected to be a neutral provider of information. However, one scholarly work has revealed that ultrasound technicians are not always that neutral.[37] The ultrasound moment marks an important transition for a woman. She has now become an expectant mother and there are strong societal expectations of how that experience should be conducted and how a woman should react to that experience. When the technician judges Juno, she has preventing her from enjoying the bonding moment, even though in her case, by giving up the baby for adoption, it is questionable whether she should even have a bonding moment. The entire ultrasound experience in *Juno* seems outside the normal mode. A completely contrary depiction of the ultrasound moment occurs in *Sex and the City* when Miranda has to "fake a sonogram" because she does not become excited by the image of her unborn child on the screen. Miranda is denying the expectation that she will use the sonogram to bond with her fetus. Later, however, viewers are reassured that Miranda has bonded with her baby when she feels the first kick and becomes touched. This is a private moment for Miranda and not shared by society.[38]

The result of the widespread depiction of ultrasound in pregnancy is that the audience is allowed to bond with the pregnancy along with the characters on the programs and films. The ultrasound experience is no longer just a private moment for the couple or the mother but a time to revel in the pregnancy and to accede to the societal expectations and ideology of what it means to be an expectant mother or father. The ideology includes excitement about the baby, the fact that any anxiety expressed is overcome by the end of an episode and by bonding early to the fetus. The ultrasound moment is not private to the character or even, in the case of Kelly Ripa, to the real-life expectant mother, but shared by all. Thus the ultrasound moment has become just another part of celebrity culture and the culture of consumption. The sonogram is now consumed readily by audiences hungry for more mediated images of their celebrities and their characters. In fact, Tom Cruise claims that the reason he bought his personal ultrasound machine when his wife Katie Holmes was pregnant was not just so that he could look at the baby any time he wanted but in order to retain and control the image. The Internet is full of offers (both real and fake) of people ready to cell images of the fetuses of celebrities. GoldenPalace.com claims they paid $3,800 for an ultrasound of Brad Pitt and Angelina Jolie's baby.[39]

Monstrous Births: Then and Now

The idea of monstrous births or pregnancy being connected with fear was common in 18th- and 19th-century medical texts. Little was known about pregnancy during this period. Pregnancy seemed scary to some and magical to others. It is unsurprising then, that some scholars suggest that these monstrous births reflect a public fearful of the unborn and the unknown.[40] Yet the monstrous birth did not go away in 20th-century America. *Rosemary's Baby* and *Alien* are two films that present pregnancy itself as something to fear. The plot of *Alien* involves trying to find a way to destroy the alien fetus that has been implanted.[41] Film critics and scholars have analyzed this film at length. Some even see it as an abortion parable in that most of the film is about trying to rid the astronaut of this creature inside of her, despite the fact that the creature's "real" mother is pleading for the creature to be saved.[42] In *Rosemary's Baby*, the title character endures a horrific pregnancy, worried about her health, and her mysterious neighbors, only to give birth to a baby that is Satanic.[43] In other films, the focus is on new babies that are mutant or monsters, such as *Eraserhead*.[44] These films reflect the 20th-century fears of pregnancy and parenthood. These are fears that any new parent today should be able to easily recognize. For example, there is the fear that the baby will take over the lives of the parents, which of course is true in many ways. There is also the fear of taking responsibility for the care of the child, the concern that the baby will "kill" us creatively, and the fear that parents will be turned into sleepless zombies. The commonality of these films and others like them is that the pregnancy and the baby are something to be feared and something that is out of the control of the characters in the plot. We still have pregnancy in jeopardy in the 21st century, but now the focus has shifted to the concern for the pregnant characters and the fear that the pregnancy will not happen.

J. J. Abrams has gained popularity for his popular television programs, including *Alias,* and *Lost* filled with characters who verbalize their feelings while in situations that are beyond their control. These shows also demonstrate his focus and fascination with pregnancy. *Alias* involved a female spy named Sydney Bristow and was played by Jennifer Garner. Toward the end of the show's run, Garner became pregnant. Rather than hide the pregnancy, Abrams made pregnancy a central component of the series. The pregnancy does not change the rugged and dangerous life of secret agent Sydney Bristow. In fact, her pregnancy becomes a part of her famous disguises.

In *Alias,* the pregnant woman is a risk taker.[45] The potential jeopardy to her baby, while ever-present throughout the program, is not attributed to Sydney herself. It is always a group of people after her that are threatening the lives of Sydney and her unborn child. At one point she is kidnapped and she worries that strange experiments are being done on her although it turns out that it is simply a lifesaving operation for the baby. The program thus reflects the conflict the woman faces versus the medical establishment. Sydney fears prenatal medical intervention by begging and threatening the surgeons not to "touch my baby" since she prefers a natural, nonintervening birth. When she is forced to give birth outside the hospital on her own, with her father and her estranged and somewhat evil mother helping her, she ends up receiving her desired natural childbirth.[46] The baby is fine at the end and she relishes in her moment of new motherhood.

Alias even explores Sidney's maternity leave and her desire to go back to work. The government provides a special nanny team of highly trained men to protect and take care of her baby. The child care represented here is a utopian and fantasy vision of the perfect child care solution for the pregnant woman. No longer is the baby a threat to the lives of the pregnant woman but instead, the baby is a welcome addition who does not impact her life negatively in any way. *Alias* represents the fantasy of the mother who can have it all. Yes, you can have a baby and be a secret agent too!

Lost involves the survivors of a plane crash and how they deal with their survival on a mysterious island. A common theme runs throughout the program. The characters have landed on an island where the current inhabitants referred to as "the others" have a problem in that nobody has ever successfully given birth to a baby conceived on the island. In fact, a fertility doctor has been brought in by "the others "to help solve the problem. It happens that one of the plane crash survivors, a character named Clair, is pregnant and is kidnapped so that the "others" can do experiments on her and prepare to possibly steal her baby. The baby is saved but the concern is ever-present. Later another character, Sun Kwon, discovers she is pregnant and she is worried over the safety of her child because of the island's problems with pregnancy. On this island pregnancy is a rare and valuable commodity to protect. Like *Alias, Lost* attributes danger not from the baby or parents, but outside forces, including the island itself and its inhabitants. These forces jeopardize the fetus and the dreams of motherhood.

Feature films have mirrored this shift in television.[47] In the film *Children of Men,* pregnancy is the central component of the plot as the end of human life is foreseen.[48] The plot involves the transfer of a lone secret pregnant woman to a safe place to protect her and the baby and to preserve life for the world. The woman's life is in jeopardy throughout the film and other characters need to sacrifice their lives for the survival of her and the infant. The hero must get the mother away to safety because the establishment wants to study her pregnancy to save mankind. The hero, and of course the audience in support, would rather she be left alone, presumably to enjoy a natural childbirth. There are echoes here from the conflict depicted in *Alias* and *Lost* over nature versus technology. This is a conflict between allowing a pregnancy to proceed on a natural course versus the need to study and thus interfere with the pregnancy. Likewise, in the film *Legion* (2009), Charlie, a pregnant waitress, needs to be protected so she can give birth to her unborn child. Pregnancy becomes an important commodity to protect, not just for the mother of the child, but for the future of the world.[49]

What all these latest programs illustrate is a shift in how producers, writers, and directors think of pregnancy. At first pregnancy and impending parenthood is something to be feared as evidenced by the actual monsters that are growing in the women's womb that come out to torture the mother and other characters surrounding her. If one could explain the 18th- and 19th-century preoccupation with pregnancy as something to feared because of the unknown, then the opposite may hold true with 20th-century depictions of pregnancy. Pregnancy is still feared despite the fact that more is known about pregnancy and the life of a fetus than ever before. The birth control pill became readily available in 1960 and abortion became legally available throughout the country with the Supreme Court's decision in 1973 in *Roe v. Wade.* Although widely debated in religious and secular circles these events were significant as a public acknowledgement that not all babies are wanted. We watch these films and programs with their "monster babies" and wrestle with the idea that perhaps not all baby births should be treated as a blessing. One can also equate the increased use of medical technology such as ultrasounds with the rising fear that a baby is an alien invading the mother's womb. Making a child into a monster also reflects a new parental anxiety about the overwhelming needs of their new baby. At the same time there has been a rise of competing books from experts on how to raise children. With this increased social and visual pressure, it is no wonder that there is both a visual apprehension about what to expect from this new life-form in the mother's body and a psychological fear over the expectations of society in how to care for this new being.

At the dawn of the 21st century the focus of this fear has shifted. Instead of the baby jeopardizing those around it, many fear they won't get pregnant in the first place. This fear makes sense considering the social context surrounding reproduction fears and technology in the 21st century. Women are waiting longer to have children, leading to rising infertility difficulties. Magazines, television programs, and news segments taunt women by asking if they are waiting too long to have children. An *Oprah* episode with Martha Stewart's daughter Alexis was devoted to women having to go through extraordinary efforts to have children. Alexis described how she spent over $28,000 per month on fertility treatments. An entire industry is now devoted to getting women pregnant. But at the same time, more technology brings more problems. In the past if you could not have children, then barring adoption, a couple's sad fate ended there. Now, lives and finances are overtaken by tests procedures, and the loss of control becomes inevitable as couples turn their bodies over to the medical profession. It seems natural then, that the focus of fear would now be of a world where women cannot get pregnant. In many parts of Europe now, the birth rates have decreased to such a low level as to become alarming to many countries.[50] Accordingly, new incentives have been adopted to encourage women to have children. Twenty-first century fictional depictions now reflect a world consumed with trying to have children, or of the consequences of not having them.

Pregnancy as Sacrifice

While monster babies may be an extreme representation of the sacrifices pregnancy brings, other films show sacrifice by focusing on the psyche of expectant couples. In these films, pregnancy precipitates choices of self-sacrifice in preparation for parenthood. A half-century ago, this burden fell largely to women as they chose motherhood or career. The 1964 Warner Brothers film *Kisses for My President* starred Polly Bergen as the first female president who runs into all sorts of problems balancing her family responsibilities with being the leader of the free world.[51] Ultimately, she resigns when she finds out that she is pregnant, a not-unexpected outcome during an era that celebrated the stay-at-home mom and hid pregnancy from public life.

In later decades, films shifted their focus to the sacrifices expectant fathers faced during pregnancy. The 1988 film *She's Having a Baby* shows a husband making adjustments to his life to get his wife pregnant and prepare for family life.[52] An unpleasant, dangerous birth scene at the end of the film makes him realize that his sacrifices were minor in comparison, and he regrets his anxiety. *Parenthood* (1989) focuses on the challenges the father faces in raising his family and his nervousness about his wife's pregnancy.[53] *Fools Rush In* (1997) also features a father's life changes as he adjusts to the family of his pregnant girlfriend.[54] Even the animated film *Shrek the Third* (2007) highlights the sacrifices of fatherhood, as Shrek adjusts to life with children.[55]

Many of these films continue to glorify pregnancy and childbirth while exploring the sacrifices of parents-to-be. The 2012 comedy *What to Expect When You're Expecting* follows five couples through their pregnancies.[56] It attempts to show the downside of pregnancy with Wendy, a baby-obsessed owner of a breast-feeding supply store, who has trouble getting pregnant. She is thrilled when she finally conceives, but she soon finds that her pregnancy symptoms do not conform to the pregnancy glow. She compares her experience to the idealized pregnancy of her "step-mother-in-law," whom she resents. The penultimate moment of the film occurs when Wendy delivers a lecture to an audience about pregnancy. She provides a wake-up call: "I'm calling bullshit on the whole thing," she rants. "Pregnancy sucks. Making a human being sucks." Her tirade, captured on video, makes her an Internet sensation and brings new customers to her store. Despite this moment of subversion, the film returns to the theme of glorifying pregnancy and childbirth, glossing over Wendy's near-death experience during childbirth and having her proclaim about her baby, "He's my glow.

He's my perfect, perfect glow." Thus, while promotional trailers for the film purport to reveal the unspoken truths about pregnancy, it ultimately praises the experience by portraying characters consumed by their pregnancies and showing the pregnancy rituals they perform. It concludes that their sacrifices were all worth it when they encountered the magical moment of holding a baby in their arms.

The 2009 film *Away We Go* introduces an expectant couple trying to find a perfect home to raise their child.[57] Their cross-country trek introduces them, and the audience, to differing parenting styles and notions of what a family is. However, the film reinforces the importance of having children and, in particular, bearing them. One couple they visit has adopted many children and seemingly has a full family life, yet they break down in grief when they discuss their infertility, demonstrating a psychological obstacle to their happiness. This scene allows the main characters to realize their fortune that they have attained a biological pregnancy. Instead of sacrifices, the film highlights the choices the characters consider regarding the family they are about to begin. *Friends with Kids* (2011) portrays sacrifice as inevitable but worth it as two friends try to avoid the pitfalls their friends have suffered with pregnancy and parenthood.[58] A promotional movie poster highlights the theme of sacrifice with check boxes offering: Love, Happiness, or Kids, with instructions to "Pick Two."

These films mirror the historical and social changes women and families have undergone. At the birth of the feminist movement, films portrayed women facing the difficult choice between family and career. As more two-income families emerged during the 1980s, fathers became more involved with family life, and films of the time reflected their impending sacrifice. Now, many films show couples negotiating together how they will face this sacrifice. However, by offering a happy ending when the baby arrives, these films minimize a real problem. Arlie Russell Hochschild defines "the second shift" as the significant amount of household and child care that women still perform even while they work outside of the home.[59] Although these films adopt the premise that the sacrifices that come with family life are shared and worth undergoing for the baby's sake, in many cases the burden of care will fall to the mother, and her sacrifice will be minimized in popular culture.

Elevator Babies: The Changing Birth Scene

Birth scenes in television and film have never been boring. Usually they are the pivotal scene of a film or television program, often during a ratings sweeps week, a season finale (or both). But a remarkable number of television characters seem about to give birth on elevators or other public places, just barely making to the hospital in time (if they do at all), when in real life most women manage to get to a hospital. These "extraordinary births" reflect the dilemmas facing producers and writers in their struggle to represent birth on television. Early television faced the challenge of how to depict a birth without actually showing what was going on in the delivery room and without offending an audience not accustomed to being allowed into a delivery room. Most of the time, the birth scenes were simply absent on television but even when they were present, it was easier to take the birth out of the delivery room. By doing so, television removed the graphic and medical aspect of the birth by making it about the mother and involving ordinary people surrounding her. In more recent years, even though depiction of birth has become a possibility, television still reflects a competing desire for a natural birth freed from technological constraints typical of modern medicine where the birth takes place in a hospital. Since having a birth at home is considered a bit too "abnormal," an extraordinary birth allows the couple on television to fulfill the desire of a "home" birth without guilt (we *tried* to get to the hospital!).[60] An exploration of the history of the birthing episodes for television programs and some films illustrate how the competition between the medicalization of birth and the alternative birth movement has impacted changes in production standards and representation of birth.

Births in the United States from the 1950s through the mid-1970s were private and closed off experiences. In some cases, even the mother did not experience the birth of her own child as she was often fully anesthetized and then later presented with her baby wrapped securely in a blanket. Certainly, the father was not allowed into the delivery room. Television producers, then, were faced with several different dilemmas concerning how to represent the birthing experience. First, in trying to mimic reality, they could not very well let viewers into a place where only expectant mothers and medical professional were permitted. The outside public had limited knowledge of the birthing experience and there was an expectation in society that the birthing experience was a private one limited to women. Accordingly, it would be offensive for family television to bring viewers inside a delivery room. The first wave of birth episodes shown on television in the 1940s through the 1960s solved these issues by placing viewers with the expectant fathers, outside the delivery room.

The father would take center stage during the birth episode, which would revolve around getting to the hospital or waiting outside the delivery room during the birth. In fact, the first television program in the United States to have a birth scene was *Mary Kay and Johnny Stearns* (1947–1950), a fictional depiction of a couple in New York City, based on the real life of a couple.[61] So, when Mary Kay became pregnant, the program's character became pregnant too. In real life, she gave birth 30 minutes before the start of the live program.[62] Not being able to show her in a delivery room, the program had the episode revolve around the father's experiences in the waiting room waiting for his wife to give birth. This set the stage for the prominence of the father in later birthing episodes. Shows often focused on the events involved in getting to the hospital and then jumped to a scene after the baby was born. *The Dick van Dyke* (1961) show's flashback episode to Ritchie's birth focuses on the fears of the father rather than the labor of the mother.[63] The parents are told by the doctor that it could be any day now. The mother is calm and does not even appear to be in labor. She is still wearing her dress and pearls and making breakfast for her husband, although she displays a pregnant bump. The episode focuses on the father's plans to get his wife to the hospital in time for the baby. He has all these plans and stays dressed in his suit to be ready. He calls a cab to have it ready just in case something happens to his car. The program's depiction of pregnancy ends with her heading to the hospital in a laundry van ("we pick up and deliver" is their motto). Now in the present, her son asks her what her favorite part of his birth was and she says that the best part was when she woke up in the hospital and he was lying down next to her. But it is apparent that everyone has missed the actual birth—not only the viewers and the father but also the mother who appears to have been anesthetized during labor. The one thing missing from Ricky's birthday is his birth! Similarly, the famous birth scene in *I Love Lucy* has them doing practice runs to the hospital. Again, the focus is on getting to the hospital—not what actually goes on in the hospital. In *Bewitched,* the baby is born within the first few minutes of the program, with those minutes being consumed with frantic Darrin rushing calm Samantha to the hospital. Then, Darrin is nervously pacing the hospital corridors while waiting for the news. The news is eventually given to him by his mother-in-law who, because she is a witch, had the privilege of secretly being present for the birth. Her presence highlights the fact that so few people, outside of the medical professionals, were able to experience the birth. Samantha is then seen primping herself before seeing her husband and then expressing disappointment that she has hardly seen the baby, not mentioning the birth at all.[64] The birth does not seem to matter here, no one asks her about it—it's all about the end result: the baby. The control over the birthing experience is reflecting a period of time when the medicalization of birth consumed the process. The message is to be sure you can get to the hospital because you don't want to risk a home birth, which of course was the norm less than two generations earlier.

By the 1970s, viewers are first beginning to view birth experiences that actually take place in the hospital. The pain of childbirth is still presented as an important experience but the significance of having the father by her side is important too. While only 15 percent of men were attending births in the late 1960s, by the late 1970s, it was more commonplace for men to be not only present for the birth but also involved in supporting the mother, and even cutting the cord.[65] *All in the Family* illustrates this moment in transition for the father as he starts to become involved in the delivery of the baby. The participation of the father at this point is still relegated to the preparation and the moment of delivery—not the entire pregnancy like it is today. Mike has plans to be a "modern" husband and expectant father and to help Gloria in the delivery room. However, he becomes nervous about it and the episodes reveal his conflict. In the episode "Mike's Pains," Archie asks him, "You are going to be in there watching a terrible thing like that?" Mike says that he isn't sure he wanted to be in the delivery room and Gloria becomes angry at him for just getting her pregnant and not supporting her in the labor room.[66] Mike represents the transition male of this period. Archie is still firmly rooted in the medical establishment. On the other hand Mike wants to be involved but still reverts at times to patriarchy. When Edith talks about the birth of her own daughter, which she saw only through the eyes of her doctor, Mike tells Gloria "If you're going to see that baby's birth in somebody's eyes, I want them to be mine." In the episode before the birth episode Mike reviews all of the breathing exercises and how he plans to keep Gloria relaxed during delivery so she will not focus on the pain.[67] Mike has his own goodie bag with snacks for himself, a rolling pin for Gloria's back, and a paper bag in case of hyperventilation. Mike plans to be a participatory father. The birth episode teases the viewers by having Gloria stuck in a phone booth, a nod to the extraordinary births often seen on television, but she still manages plenty of time to make it to the hospital room. The episode also teases us by showing Mike in the traditional role of the nervous father panicking when Gloria actually goes into labor. He forgets phone numbers that he always knew and keeps stammering, unable to complete a sentence. In the labor room, Gloria does not seem to be in a lot of pain in the beginning and they both seem tired of waiting for the baby to arrive. But once they are actually in the hospital, Michael is calm again, working as coach and telling her to push and counting for her. He is so proud of his wife and says, "She's sitting here panting and pushing and

making jokes" and the nurse tells him to keep calm but in reality, in comparison to previous fathers, he's the ideal participatory father. He says it
wasn't too bad, and she answers, "Not with you here to help."[68] The father
gains some of the credit in this birth and this is an important step in moving the birthing process away from being a private experience to becoming
a more shared public experience.

From the 1980s through today, a father is expected in the delivery room
and the comedy arises from the obstacles they face in trying to be there.
The challenges fathers face are no longer coming from the medical establishment or from societal expectations for fathers to be separated from
the birthing process. Instead, television represents the challenges as being
physical obstacles in the husband trying to reach his wife. In the *Friends* first
birth episode (where Ross becomes a father when his lesbian ex-wife gives
birth), he is unable to get to the birth because he is accidentally locked in
a supply cabinet.[69] In the *Mad About You* episode where Jamie gives birth,
she is in the hospital waiting for Paul who is locked out of the hospital
because of a film shoot going on there. Half the episode focuses on his attempts to reach her. Part of the humor of the episode rests in the reversal
of the typical experience of the mother unable to get there.[70] But you also
see here an important shift in the expectations of an audience that now
expects the father to be at the bedside of the mother. The 1980s program,
Thirtysomething has an episode that portrays the birth experience of Susan-
nah and Gary but where the focus in on Gary.[71] In fact, the doctor takes him
aside to tell him that he needs to do something to help progress the labor.
Similarly, the importance of the father in the birth scene becomes truly
vivid with the film *Father of the Bride Part II,* where the father has both
a pregnant wife and a pregnant daughter (whose husband is not there at
first) and he's trying to juggle both rooms, trying to support everyone.[72] In
Knocked Up, the father is at his most responsible, calm, and collected self
when she is ready to give birth. He takes control, resolves a fight between
his girlfriend and her doctor, and then actually kicks out her sister (who
was supposed to be her labor coach) to assert his place in the room and
his position in the family. In today's birthing episodes, it seems that the
more people involved in the birth, the better the television experience. For
example, in *7th Heaven* (aired in 2005), Lucy has her baby unexpectedly in
an elevator. Her brother, who is in medical school, is there to assist her but
both of them (and particularly Lucy's husband) are grossed out about the
idea of her brother viewing her private area.[73] But, when she comes out the
whole family is waiting. Much of the humor of the birth episode of *How I
Met Your Mother* is focused on the fact that Marshall is out of town on a

trip that she forced him on because *he* was becoming too obsessed with the birth. Throughout the birth, she keeps asking for him, screaming, "Where the hell is Marshall? I can't do this without Marshall."[74] This becomes an interesting moment, as women in previous time periods birthed with only other women present, but now fathers have become an integral part of the process.

On nonfiction programs, like *A Baby Story,* the birthing scene is the climactic moment in each episode. Although it is a documentary and depicts real life the show must still conform to the standards of television. In order to be interesting and easy to produce, each episode has to have a typical storyline and there needs to be some conflict. Since all the families are chosen as representatives of nice couples who are in love and have few problems but are about to give birth, the conflict has to happen in the birth itself where it is the woman battling nature in order to give birth. The show shifts its focus suddenly from calm parents discussing their excited expectations of giving birth to suddenly having the mother in pain and trying to deal with the birth and her family members coping with seeing her in pain. Conflict appears as the parents have to cope with unexpected decisions about such things as pain medication or unexpected cesareans. Because the audience is allowed in as a witness to the birth, the birth experience becomes public, and not just because there are extended relatives popping in to share this event. Fictional depictions of birth have also started to show more relatives in the birthing room. In *Mad About You,* Jamie surrounds herself with as many women in her life as possible in order for the experience to be meaningful to her as a moment where she is being welcomed into a club of sorts. This scene is reminiscent of early birthing periods when it was the women in the community, not the doctors, who help the women through the process. In the birth scene of their friends, the characters in *Notes from the Underbelly* gather together to support their friend in labor whose husband has not arrived yet.[75] All the friends pop in and out to visit throughout the scene and the doctor is relegated to just short visits—it is the friends who will see the mother through this experience. On television, the doctors are starting to play less of a role, only appearing for a few minutes in a scene and then at the end for the actual delivery as seen in *Knocked Up,* where the doctor ends up being mostly perceived as useless to the couple. In the birth episode of *How I Met Your Mother,* Lily is told that she cannot have an epidural, but her doctor reassures her: "Don't worry. The baby will slide right out. It's like a whoosh, like a water slide. A slightly painful waterslide." In a similar metaphor in the *Up All Night* birth scene, Reagan, when about to start pushing, warns the doctor "I think this baby is going to shoot out like a cannon ball."[76] Much of the humor of the program comes in the contrast in these statements with the reality of the births, which are both presented as painful, with *Up All Night* ending in a cesarean section. The modern-day birth, then, presents the mother, father, and people she chooses to surround herself with as being in control over the birthing process rather than the medical establishment, although the hospital is still generally seen as the place to have the baby. It is best to be in a hospital just in case something goes wrong, and on television, the conflict often comes from when it does.[77] Despite the increased presence of people in the birth scene, however, viewers are still left retaining the mystery of childbirth.

In a critic's review, Neil Genzingler discusses recent television episodes that feature births, most showing the women in agonizing pain or in extraordinary circumstances. He also writes of at least two shows that have women and doctors referring to the vaginal area as "down there."[78] In the birth episode in *Parenthood*, Christina is brought to the hospital by her brother-in-law and warns him not to look "down there."[79] Similarly, during a birth scene of the show *Up All Night*, viewers watch Reagan and Chris react with revulsion when offered a mirror to watch the baby crowning. Although viewers are invited into the birth scene, they are reminded that there are parts of birth that should stay hidden.

Conclusions

If you were to try to understand pregnancy in the mid-20th century by watching television, you would probably think that babies are immaculately conceived, delivered by stork, and fathers were bumbling fools. Because the public thought pregnancy was a private subject, television producers curtailed its depiction. The announcement of a baby on a television show seemed to be a surprise to all its characters. Rather than consulting medical professionals, *I Love Lucy* relied on a team of clergy to advise producers on how to represent this delicate subject.[80] Deliveries simply were not shown on television.

By the 1970s and 1980s, film and television still did not reveal much about how babies were conceived, but fictional fathers were more involved and necessary to the process, and one could watch women heroically deliver their babies both inside and outside the delivery room. From the 1990s to today, much of the secret side of pregnancy has been exposed. Getting pregnant is as important as the pregnancy itself for most programs, and infertility has become an essential part of many plots. Watch the program *Knocked Up* in theatres and witness everything from the conception of the baby to morning sickness, pregnant sex, and the delivery. Review pregnancy on film and television, and you see how pregnancy has been transformed from a delicate private subject to a detailed public discussion. Gone are the days when the delivery scene is no longer the first moment when we get to meet the little one since this happens as early as the sonogram. We now even see a chemical representation of the baby as we look at the pregnancy sticks that the characters brandish as if they were popsicles. Pregnancy is not only visible, but also fashionable. Today, pregnancy is a subject that has moved beyond fictional depiction; reality television stars like Tori Spelling routinely show off and discuss in detail their pregnancies.

As pregnancy is routinely featured in popular culture, it is only natural to cover what comes afterward: the birth. However, thanks to television, decency standards regarding nudity and advertiser and public disinterest in seeing graphic depictions of childbirth, television and film birth scenes generally focus on friends, family, and manufactured comic or suspenseful plotlines that surround the birth event. This means that a key aspect of childbirth, how the baby actually comes out, often is missing. Funmilayo Brown, the executive director of Choices in Childbirth, has become concerned about the social and political ramifications of these missing representations. The women she meets while she reaches out to inform them about their options during childbirth often do not think about labor and birth until they are at least halfway through their pregnancies. Brown describes this as an experience that is unique to American culture; around the world, greater access to midwives and natural birthing allows more opportunities for women to witness birth by the time they are ready to have their own baby. She is dismayed by television images that present birth only as an emergency. "It's not very good that we don't have some understanding of this process, this very natural, clear process, that we all go through to be born," she laments. "It's crazy when you think about it." Brown herself experienced what happens when a culture lacks this crucial information. "When I was in labor and walking through the Village on my way to St. Vincent's," she said, "people thought I was dying. Someone even called 911, and an ambulance showed up on 13th Street ready to take me to 12th Street." While popular culture offers far more representations of pregnancy and birth today, these representations are still limited, and these limitations have the power to discourage women from fully comprehending and preparing for childbirth. Pregnancy and childbirth have come out of the delivery room, but for popular culture, what happens inside the delivery room is still largely a mystery.

Chapter 5

The Backseat Pregnancy

When my pregnant sister walked into her kitchen one day, she noticed that her husband had set aside a little dish filled with sesame seeds, nuts, and fruits. She asked her husband, "What is this all about?" and he said that it was related to the e-mails that she was sending him. Each week, she would forward him an e-mail from one of the baby forums that she subscribed to that told her how the baby was progressing. "This week, your baby is the size of a sesame seed, next week a cherry, next week a nut, next week an avocado." He decided to collect the things that the baby was supposed to resemble so that he could look at its progress each day.

This worked for about a month until the cleaning lady came in one day and accidentally disposed of "their baby." But her husband's effort to visualize the baby is nothing to laugh about. For a woman, tracking a baby's progress is an internal experience. Even before a mother begins to feel a baby's movements (toward the end of the second trimester or beginning of the third) her every craving, mood swing, or twinge is a reminder that there is a baby inside. On the other hand, men experience a pregnancy secondhand.

Couvade syndrome describes men who experience symptoms similar to the woman during pregnancy.[1] As far back as 260 BC, there were records of men who would lie in bed with pregnancy symptoms while women would take care of them. These practices continued for some time and are still practiced today in some parts of the world. Scholars and scientists have all offered different reasons for why men would want or need to experience their wives' pregnancy. Some offer a biological explanation, while Freudians explain it as an embodiment of psychological envy of the woman's condition. Other writers offer reasons that are more spiritual or societal in nature. All agree, however, that there have always been men that have had some type of significant involvement in pregnancy.[2] In contemporary

United States, men have manifested Couvade through feelings of fatigue, weight gain, or even morning sickness. These men often treat these effects as something to joke or brag about. For example, if you check out YouTube today, a popular photo image or montage is the paired photo of a husband and wife, with the wife actually pregnant and the husband sporting his own "sympathy weight" of an extra 30 pounds in his belly. Men are working harder than before to get as close to the pregnancy as possible. For some men, a woman is only a necessary womb but not an emotional part of the pregnancy. Changing family structures, perspectives on feminism, and the role of marketers to help create a new type of involved dad are just some factors that contribute to this shift. However, the strongest factor that allows men to participate in pregnancies in a new and deeper manner is the advance in medical technology.

The Male Ticking Clock

If you ask men whose wives had babies before the 1970s, most of them can tell you the exact moment when their wife came to them and told them that she was having a baby. For many of these men, there was also an element of surprise in finding out this news. While men were certainly involved in conceiving a baby, they did not involve themselves in verifying whether conception had occurred. If you talk to men now, however, you will find that conception is now a shared experience. As a result of advances in technology and changes in the societal expectations of men and women, men are now involved in the whole process of preparing for conception rather than just the act itself. Additionally, pregnancy tests, now easily done at home, are a shared experience for the man and the woman. There is even a new iPod application called "PMS buddy," which enables men to track their wife's or girlfriend's period, ostensibly to better cope with their mood swings. This new technology also helps men to be in touch with their partners' ovulation cycles. With just a little math men can figure out when it's best to conceive (or not conceive). This is just one way that men are taking ownership of the fertility process.

Prehistoric men were once so far removed from the fertility process that they had no idea of their role in getting women pregnant in the first place.[3] Due to the length of time between sex and a visible pregnancy, people did not make the connection between the two. In the Paleolithic and Neo-Paleolithic periods, the mother goddess figure is prevalent. People believed that women alone were responsible for getting pregnant, and consequently for taking care of the child that resulted. Even when men began to understand that there was a menstrual cycle, they did not track their partners' cycles or connect them to conception or pregnancy.[4]

Over the course of time, scientific advances and societal changes began to bring men into the process. For example, the Ancient Greek concept of citizenship was connected to lineage and legitimacy. Men therefore became newly vested in making sure that they had biological ties to their offspring.[5] This caused men to segregate women and idealize chastity. On the other hand, men remained out of touch with the inner workings of a woman's body.

Modern technology now gives men opportunities to not only become familiar with their wives' menstrual cycles but also to assist in its "control." Mike, one husband I spoke with, describes how he took over the conception process from his wife when the couple faced difficulties conceiving. He asked his wife for the dates of her last periods, did some research online, and created his own Excel spreadsheet that he used to figure out their ideal days to conceive. Websites like Go28days.com allow anyone to monitor a monthly cycle and to learn which dates bear maximum chances of conception. Inventions like the ovulation test kit and the pregnancy test kit have also moved the conception process from a mystery to a transparent science. Women are now able to predict their cycle through self-examination, while men can join in the process by examining women's cycles and planning the best days of conception.

These technologies have taken on a particular importance in recent times. As more women have deferred having children until later in life, when conception is more difficult, their partners have taken a more extensive role regarding conception. Sometimes the process is uncomfortable as men have to donate sperm in order for it to be screened for virility or to be used for fertilization or in vitro. Even when men remain in the backseat, they are nevertheless along for the ride. They give hormone injections, they bring their wives to doctor's visits, and they wait alongside them for the stick to change colors.

Men are starting to reference "biological clocks" of their own. On the scientific level, some recent studies actually suggest that males may have a biological clock and that the older they get, the more likely they may be to produce less healthy children. Australian researchers from the University of Queensland linked older fathers and lower IQs in children.[6] Harry Fisch, the author of the *Male Biological Clock,* warns men that they have a limit on fertility too and that older men may be more likely to produce children with certain medical problems.[7] Studies like these spark blog posts and comments about whether men feel the biological clock ticking.[8] Some say that since men have a longer time to father a child or at least a possibility to father a child, they cannot experience it in the same way. Others argue that their husbands or boyfriends are the ones pressuring them to have a child. My own interviews with pregnant women and their partners reflect that in some couples, it was the man that had the stronger desire trying to convince his wife to get pregnant.

New technology also allows men to take control of their fertility in several ways. Costs for sperm banking have come down and now men can freeze their sperm for use later. At first, this type of sperm banking was used by males who were going to anonymously donate sperm, husbands whose wives had fertility problems or men who were going to undergo some type of cancer treatment and needed to preserve their fertility. But, these days, fertility centers, capitalizing on the above studies, are after the healthy young men. The New Hope Fertility Center in New York City encourages men and women to preserve their fertility, warning men that "While men continue to regenerate new sperm throughout their lifetimes, their sperm quality begins to deteriorate after age 25."[9]

Perhaps the idea of a biological ticking clock for men needs to be expanded to the idea of a psychological clock as well. Men probably always had a desire to have a family or to put it more crudely to pass on their seed. But, these days as women are waiting longer to get pregnant because they are having their own fulfilling careers, we may be seeing men developing that desire to start a family. With the added pressure of these newer studies and fertility clinics appealing directly to them, men may face social pressure to procreate (or preserve their ability to) in ways they never had before.

As helpful as these new technologies are, they also may lead to new problems and confusion. In most cases, the couples are in agreement regarding the goals of fertility treatments. In a few cases, however, disputes occur when couples begin to disagree with each other on what to do with the embryos. For example, when the couple divorces (which is not all that uncommon as fertility treatments often strain a couple's relations), the custody of the embryo often comes into question. In 2000, a man sued his ex-wife because she was implanting embryos that contained his sperm even though he had decided that he did not want her creating children with them.[10] This law suit illustrates the confusion that begins to arise as men's role in conception begins to shift from just a sperm donor to a much more vocal and active participant in the conception process.

Now that more couples wait longer to become pregnant, they often face more difficulty conceiving. As the process moves from a private experience between couples to a scientific endeavor to get the woman pregnant, the man's part in the conception process becomes just as exposed as the woman's. Since men are sometimes the cause of the infertility, they must take tests and visit the fertility clinic. In addition, more invasive fertility procedures like in vitro fertilization break down the process, so you see more clearly the man's role versus the woman's. The male's sperm is separated from his body and combined with the woman's egg to create an embryo. But since this form of conception is out of the womb, it can shift control from a woman to a man. Women used to control the entire process because it all took place in her body. But once conception and the male's part in it is segmented, men can acquire more control over the process and can assert a legal claim over an embryo or take a greater role in the planning and timing of the conception. Thus new technology not only creates more possibilities to couples having difficulty conceiving, but also shifts the relationship and power between men and women.

Bump Envy

If one thinks about a pregnant celebrity, it doesn't take long to conjure up the famous image of Demi Moore posing for photographer Annie Leibovitz while pregnant and nude on the cover of *Vanity Fair* magazine. Less talked about, but certainly as interesting, is the *Spy Magazine* parody cover that featured a doctored photo of Bruce Willis who was Demi Moore's husband at the time also naked and pregnant. This imagined fascination with a pregnant man has a long and history. The idea of the male birth can be traced as far back as the Book of Genesis with the birth of Eve from Adam's rib. Artists and scholars have debated whether Eve should be perceived as being created by God or as a creation of Adam.

A popular fable during the Middle Ages has men fearing that they were pregnant because of a urine mishap. In one version of this story found on a Latin manuscript, Achilles believes that he is pregnant and about to die because of his inability to give birth. It is found out later that his daughter is the one pregnant and had switched her urine for a doctor's test.[11] In another version of this story, a servant comes to a house for a job and is hired by the master of the house when he promises that he has been castrated. Thus the master can have the servant sleep with his daughter and save room. The servant was lying and ends up having sex at the girl's request. The girl ends up running into a priest and convincing him to make love to her and the priest ends up with pains. In trying to give a urine sample, he has a servant handle his urine, and the servant spills it, substituting cow urine. There are lots of variations of these stories but typically, the women are blamed for desiring sex and causing the male pregnancy because of the woman's position on top during lovemaking.[12]

This motif has endured into modern times, with even the famous *Little Red Riding Hood* having been reconceptualized as a story about the wolf expecting a baby. In a 1971 and a 1989 version, the Big Bad Wolf himself becomes pregnant. In these versions of the fairy tale, a masculine, male figure of violence becomes feminized, and maternal. At the end of the story, when he devours Little Red Riding Hood he ends up with a pregnant belly and the huntsman needs to cut her out of his belly, cesarean style.[13] Therefore, throughout history stories and fables have been used to reimagine the role of men and women and to consider what the world would be like if men carried a baby.

This topic is still a favorite for entertainment today. Some iconic television programs have imagined the pregnant man as a form of comic relief. In an episode of *Bewitched*, Samantha's husband Darrin gets a spell cast upon him by his mother-in-law, a witch, to make him pregnant in order for him to become more sympathetic to his wife's pregnancy. Throughout the episode, the program shows the ridiculousness of a man being pregnant because he is unable to cope with the physical symptoms. The program was created in 1965 and reflects the contemporary view of men and women, gender roles, and women's power. Created during second-wave feminism (which would challenge and reshape the role of women, and thus men, in society), the program examines the man's and the woman's role in a relationship. As a witch, Samantha has all this power but her main goal is to serve as a good wife and mother defined by a traditional 1950s perspective. Her mother, who is also a witch, uses her power to defy traditional societal expectations of motherly roles and becomes a more subversive character, though one looked at as interfering and pesky by the other characters.

In this *Bewitched* episode, the roles of man and woman are reversed as Darrin experiences the pregnancy. Much of the humor is derived from the physical manifestations of pregnancy. Darrin walks around holding his back and yawning. Mood swings are also a part. He is completely unable to function at work. During a business meeting, all he can focus on is the food on the table. When his boss critiques him at work, Darrin becomes upset and starts crying, looking foolish and "feminine." The program ultimately returns the roles to their rightful place when Darrin's spell is lifted and he is able to assume his more natural state.[14] Here, pregnancy is not so much envied as thought of something that is burdensome and rightly belongs to the woman. The program illustrates not only what would happen if a man gets pregnant, but also what would happen to a pregnant woman trying to cope in a workplace. The program implies that the physical manifestations of pregnancy overwhelm a woman to the extent that she is unable to accomplish anything beyond maintaining her pregnancy. Pregnancy is seen here as a burden and thought of only in terms of the physical discomfort attached to it. The program uses the image of the pregnant man to imagine the danger of the proposed power for women. The program ends with Darrin returning to his rightful role as the man in the house, unburdened by pregnancy, and responsible for being caring to his wife while she is pregnant in this delicate state.

In Jacques Demy's 1973 film, *A Slightly Pregnant Man*, the main character, Marco (played by Marcello Mastroianni) finds himself pregnant. He quickly accepts the pregnancy after the doctor explains that this may be occurring due to changes in diet (hormones in chicken, perhaps) and that it is going to be the new societal trend. The film tackles the feminist and gender questions raised by the idea of a male becoming pregnant. His wife Irene (Catherine Deneuve) owns her own beauty parlor shop, and talks with her customers about how this will help men to experience what it is like to be a woman, and could change their perspectives on issues like abortion. While the film seems radical in the way that it takes on feminist issues, we find out at the end of the film that the whole thing was a mistake and that he was never pregnant at all. Furthermore, Marco accepts it easily and at the end, his wife is pregnant, returning the world to its proper social order.[15] The film seems willing to imagine but reminds the audience that it is only a fantasy.

Another "pregnant man" film is 1978's *Rabbit Test*, which takes place during the height of second-wave feminism. Directed by Joan Rivers, the film stars Billy Crystal (in his first starring role in a feature film) as a character who ends up getting pregnant. Crystal is a virgin (at least at the beginning of the film) who lives across the hall from his mother who babies him throughout the film. While the film does not really explain how he gets pregnant, it is noted that he is on the bottom when he is having sex.[16] This is reminiscent of the earlier fairytales, where this position of lovemaking is thought to cause a man to get pregnant. The person getting pregnant is considered the victim, the subject of sexual dominance. The rest of the film is about him feeling the symptoms of pregnancy, trying to have a romance, and fearing the government about to capture him for fear of what a pregnant man will do to society. Unlike Demy's film, *Rabbit Test* contains little focus on the politics of pregnancy and Crystal's character treats his pregnancy as a punishment throughout the film. While the French film

A Slightly Pregnant Man presents a man who is "man" enough to accept being pregnant, the American film presents someone who isn't man enough not to get pregnant.

In an episode of the *Cosby Show* (aired in 1989), Cliff Huxtable has a dream where he imagines all the men in the program pregnant and living the uncomfortable experience of a pregnant woman. While most critics focus on the *Cosby Show* as a breakthrough in representation of African Americans in a positive light, it also needs to be noted for its portrayal of an involved dad, who splits care of the household and children with his lawyer wife. In many episodes, the viewer frequently sees him watching the children, caring for them while they are sick, comforting them when they are upset, and being a primary caretaker. His career as an obstetrician also places him in touch with females and pregnancy on a daily basis, and the program frequently showed him in his doctor's office or hospital interacting with pregnant women.

The *Cosby* episode that features pregnant men has Cliff crossing a line into the world of women. The men walk around similar to Darrin in *Bewitched,* in discomfort and manifesting the physical pains of pregnancy. The program makes fun of pregnant women, exaggerating their inability to sit on a couch or the way their hormones prevent them from listening to logic. At the same time, though, the program critiques the male/female divide. The episode has Denise (Cliff's daughter) say about her husband, "If anyone could give him twins, it would be me," while Claire says, "I can't wait to get started on the next one."[17] The women laugh and the show is poking fun at the way the virility of men is treated when a pregnant woman is seen. The program ends with the men each giving birth to an object that is important to them. The fruits of male labor are consumer products, not something to nurture. Ultimately, the program seems to be showing the limits of men's involvement in the sphere of women.

In the 1994 film *Junior,* Arnold Schwarzenegger plays a man who becomes pregnant as a result of a science experiment. This film, unlike *Rabbit Test,* explains how he became pregnant in this experiment but the rest of the film follows the typical pattern of him experiencing the weird looks and discomfort of pregnancy. The film, like Schwarzenegger's earlier film *Kindergarten Cop,* uses the departure from his traditional action-packed film to allow the audience to relish in the humiliation of an über-masculine action star for laughs—he can defeat terrorists, but can he handle mood swings or change a diaper? This both reinforces traditional gender roles because "Arnold" looks silly in these situations but at the same time offers a new appreciation of the other.

The story archetype of the pregnant man crosses over into the realm of the real with Thomas Beatie. Transgendered, Beatie was born a woman biologically but longed to become a man. While Beatie assumed a male role socially and in his outward physical characteristics, he did not undergo a sex-change operation, with the result that he could still carry a child. Discussed in the tabloid press and then moving to the more mainstream press, he reached the peak of his popularity after appearances on Oprah Winfrey's talk show and then an interview with Barbara Walters. He said in these interviews that he chose to carry this baby but still considered himself the baby's father and his wife the mother.

Beatie encountered difficulty trying to fill out a birth certificate for his baby, as his local government did not share Beatie's more fluid conceptions of male and female, and mother and father. His critics keep trying to "out" him as a woman. Elizabeth Hasselbeck, a host on *The View,* who is known for her conservative positions, complains on the program of Beatie trying to take over the uniquely female experience of being pregnant.[18]

The reception of Beatie's story contrasts with the popularity of a fictional or comedic depiction of a pregnant man. Much of this humor in fictional male pregnancies is derived from a cross-dressing man (like the classic Milton Berle sketches) and in the programs we saw, most of them do not even result in a baby at the end. The men were simply taught a lesson by the fear and inconvenience of being pregnant. But when you have an actual man who is not simply cross-dressing for comedic effect but moving into "a woman's place," real questions are raised.

Beatie epitomizes all of these questions about the idea of mother and father as a biological versus social role. Do the social roles emerge from the biological? Does a mother naturally wake up at midnight to the cries of her baby (while her husband snores at her side) because it's a biological thing? Or, are these social roles arbitrary? Beatie's experience makes some people uncomfortable (and Hasselbeck's complaints are extremely mild if you glance at the all the blog postings about him) because he forces society to debate the idea of what is a man and a woman, and who needs to or chooses to serve what functions in society.

In the long tradition of fictional representations of pregnant men, the pregnant man is unnatural and the pregnancy is something to fear. Instead of women gaining equal power when the men are pregnant, the men are shown as unable to cope or focus on anything other than being pregnant—thus implying that a pregnant woman is not suitable for workplace functioning or other powerful and integral positions in society. In the case of Thomas Beatie, he runs into the problem of people refusing to accept him as a man because of the threat that a male pregnancy seems to pose for people.

For some feminists like Shulamith Firestone, the pregnant man could be the solution to the male/female power problem. In *The Dialectic of Sex: The Case for Feminist Revolution,* she argues that taking reproduction away from the female domain can enable women to have equal power in society, since they would not necessarily need to take time off from work to carry the child, give birth to the child, and nurse the child. The pregnant man is her utopian vision of an equal society. For Firestone, the solution seems a type of post-human society where there is little differentiation between men and women. For her, women need to be released from the burden of pregnancy.

But for others, as in the television and cinematic representations discussed above, a more realistic solution is not to try to create a new type of human but to help men to be able to feel and understand the woman's experience. The idea of male pregnancy raises these essential questions about whether the goal for society should be to try to create completely equal genders or to embrace differences. Is a biological fix (allowing men to get pregnant) going to allow a woman to break past social ideologies that keep her in "her place?"

Reality Check

Changing notions of power and pregnancy are appearing onscreen in new ways. Reflecting the increased involvement of the father in pregnancy, television programs now showcase fathers as the stars of the show, with programs that focus on their needs during this special time. The promotional images for the VH1 reality program *Scott Baio is 46 . . . and Pregnant* show a pregnant-looking Baio. A former child actor, Baio is the star of the program despite the fact that it is his model girlfriend who is actually pregnant on the show. But the program is all about *him*. It's a program, really, about impending fatherhood and his efforts to adjust to what is going to happen to him. But, paradoxically, it is actually useful because what it does is allow, possibly for the first time, an examination of the male's role in the pregnancy process. He takes a "daddy-to-be" class, where he discusses his fears about becoming a father. Even after the baby is born, he returns to the "daddy-to-be" class to inform them that he hasn't felt his nirvana. He's not thrilled and excited to be a father. He just feels like he's in the movie *Groundhog Day.*

Baio's words and sentiments are probably comforting to many new fathers who also recognize that sleeplessness feeling but wanting to feel the bonding. His show exposes the challenges and myths of pregnancy and fatherhood—all from the man's perspective. In one class Baio talks about how he truly feels like his life is "over." This conception of fatherhood is interesting because in earlier periods, the man's life wouldn't feel "over" because it was the woman who assumed the primary burden of child care. As an involved father, Baio also experiences the anxieties and sacrifices previously experienced only by mothers. Baio epitomizes this shift from stud to father and illustrates the sacrifice of male involvement. Yet, despite the fact that his show sounds similar to other reality shows that focus on new mothers (those on TLC like *A Baby Story* or *Bringing Baby Home*), Baio's show is different because instead of garnering much sympathy, he comes across as self-absorbed, narcissistic, and whiny. This is partly because of his persona but perhaps the idea of a pregnancy show focused solely on the male perspective might also be challenging viewer expectations and tolerance.

Another reality program features former *Saved by the Bell* star Mario Lopez in the VH1 program *Saved by the Baby*.[19] In the various episodes Mario struggles with the fact that he has to share pregnancy decisions with his wife, Courtney. In one scene, they are waiting at the doctor's office for an ultrasound while arguing over whether to find out the sex of the baby. Courtney says to the cameras about their disagreement "It's really been bothering me because I want to know what's inside of me." Mario tells her "If God wanted you to know, he would have made a window." When the doctor comes in and asks Courtney how she is feeling, Mario answers in place of her, and Courtney makes the doctor clarify that he was asking about her. Then, they bring their fight to the doctor, who Mario tries to convince to be on his side about not finding out the sex. However, the doctor sides with Courtney saying, "She has all the power here because she's carrying the baby." This scene would seem ludicrous to women of previous centuries, who would have had full access to the knowledge of the pregnancy (without the involvement of the father) and then would need to cede control to men once the baby was born. Contrary to the doctor's beliefs, Courtney no longer has all the power. In fact Mario wins this round and they do not find out the sex of the baby. Later, Mario also is making a decision about not circumcising the baby (if it's a boy) and Courtney says, "I have no say in the matter." Mario appears overly involved, but it is attributed more to his controlling personality (in one scene they compare his fastidious closet with his baby decision making) than to changes in how pregnancy is perceived these days. The rest of the program deals with his transition to fatherhood as he tries to balance his work, his friends, and his new roles of fatherhood, even wondering whether he will be on time for the birth. His wife has become a more minor character, despite the fact that she is the one carrying the baby.

The premise for the entire film *Due Date* is about a prospective father trying to make it home in time for the birth of his child.[20] The film pairs two opposite figures, showcasing the responsible nature of the expectant father by contrasting him with a childlike, pure "id" type figure. Yet, the pulling of the heartstrings of the film work because of the viewer's supposed knowledge that this is an involved father who has clearly been vested and involved in the pregnancy. Other programs, such as *Dad Camp* on VH1 is all about transforming what the VH1 blog describes as "preparing six young men headed down the road to deadbeat fatherhood" to become good fathers. The program's theme rests in the assertion that, even before the baby is born, there are expectations of what it means to be a good expectant father and that the role these men play now could determine their future relationships with their children.[21] These programs represent a shift from previous times when not only was the mother the central star but births were also the most important moment (aside from conception) for the fathers. As these shows illustrate, these days it is just the culmination of months of activity and preparation.

The Daddy Blog

Google the phrase "fathers-to-be and pregnancy" and the first hit you reach is the blog, www.HisBoysCanSwim.com. This blog (which also links to a Twitter account) is an anonymous accounting of a pregnancy from both the prospective father and mother, pseudonymously called "Tarzan" and "Jane." Tarzan created the blog as a present for his wife when he found out she was pregnant. He thought she would enjoy the experience of documenting her pregnancy, and he chimes in with his own entries. The blog is so popular that it receives 1,000–2,000 hits a day, while the associated Twitter account has 13,500 followers. Since this is an anonymous website, these readers and followers are all strangers to the authors, and this fan base has grown as the authors have received publicity for their website and links from other websites. Tarzan was surprised by the fact that its followers are not just pregnant women and dads-to-be but also grandparents, and parents who lived through the process years earlier. Also, there are a group of nonpregnant people who are just interested in the experience.

Tarzan's entries are important to him because of both his desire to document the pregnancy for their future baby ("Baby Tarzan as he is known in the blogosphere) and also because of he has found that few men are included in the pregnancy experience. Tarzan described to me his first experience at the doctor's office: "I'm 99% of the time, the only guy there. I'm sitting in the waiting room surrounded by women magazines. There's no magazines there for guys. I guess doctors don't expect it or just doesn't happen that often. Every single magazine is all women gossip magazines and girl magazines. I sit in there and just play games on my cellphone. I can only remember one, maybe two times, there was another guy in the room." He was disappointed by how little knowledge he was able to gain from his friends: "One of my guy friends just had a baby. He never talked to me about any of this and I'm sure he went through the pregnancy hormones and I never heard about any of this from any guy friends. Guys—for whatever reason, keep it hidden and don't like to talk about it."

Tarzan was interested in expressing the pregnancy experience from the male perspective. Some of his blogs have been about his helplessness as a prospective father. One blog entry from Tarzan, 14 weeks into the pregnancy, reads like this: "I feel so bad for her. I feel so helpless. I don't know what to do. I really hope this will pass soon because I couldn't stand seeing Jane get sick all throughout her pregnancy. The biggest reason I hope this nausea passes is because I want my fun, happy, energetic Jane back, and I want her to feel good more than anything else."

But Tarzan is also trying to reorient the experience to be one that a male can enjoy. Although Jane offered to include him in the baby shower, she says Tarzan was not interested. "He thought it was way more girly than he wanted to be involved in." Instead, Tarzan is working to "masculinize" other parts of the pregnancy. For example, he redesigned the ubiquitous weekly e-mail updates that describe the fetus's development in the womb to be more relatable to men. For week 7, for example, he writes, "Your baby is the size of the power button on your TV remote." In another weekly update, he compares the size of the baby to the head of a hammer. In week 16, the baby is the size of a small stud finder. He saves the best for last: "Pregnancy Week 37: Your baby is the size of the electric motor in the $110,000 2008 Tesla which can go from 0 to 60 in 3.9 seconds. Sweet."

Even Tarzan's pseudonym emphasizes this masculine perspective and experience. This is an important illustration of how pregnancy has shifted from a medicalized female experience to a more social one in which men can participate. Perhaps the name is a reassurance that his is not one of those overtly touchy feely perspectives but a more macho one. Tarzan is using his website as a way to become involved in the process and assert his presence not only to his future child but also to a world in which men are more and more welcomed into the process. A blog posting in Jane's 38th week reads like this:

> I'm ready to become a father. Huh. It's a whole new me saying that. Maybe it's the class we went to and some videos we've watched. Maybe it's books we've read. Maybe it's blogging about the pregnancy journey. Maybe it's reading all of the comments people like you make on our posts. Maybe it's everything combined. Maybe it's watching Jane through her 9 months of pregnancy. Whatever it is that has prepared me, *I feel like I'm ready now.*

I'll See You in the Delivery Room

In the history of men's involvement with their partners' pregnancies, time and location have been major factors. If one traces certain patterns across evolutionary periods, one finds that generally males spent more time mating than nurturing pregnant mates. Some believe that the explanation to this may be a biological one, as males have an unconscious urge to pass on their genetics and need to focus on mating as much as possible to make sure that happens. This theory further maintains that while females are sure that the child they are carrying is genetically related to them, males can never be sure, with the result that it makes more practical sense for them to continue to mate rather than to remain with the child and nourish him or her. Sarah Hrdy's well-known studies on primates illustrate the quandary that males face. With no obvious sign of ovulation, simian primates can never be sure that the offspring belongs to them. Hrdy offers the explanation that this fact may stem from a survival tactic—since the offspring's biological father cannot be proven, other males with which a mother may have mated would be less likely to harm the offspring post-birth.[22] But this has never been true for all primates, as male Titi monkeys are typically monogamous and other males do bond with the infants.[23]

Tracing the history of male involvement among humans, you find similar patterns in that historically, most men were not very involved in nurturing their offspring but that there have been cases where there has been male involvement. Anthropologist Richard Reed has investigated pregnancy and childbirth practices from the perspective of men by interviewing men across the world. His historical as well as his more recent research illustrates places and times in which men have connected with women during pregnancy. Reed describes the Couvade experience, when men display pregnancy symptoms, as playing an important role in pregnancy throughout the world. The work of anthropologist Alan Holmberg documents the

Siriono of Bolivia, where the men are responsible for birthing the soul of the babies and thus must abstain from certain foods and practices during the pregnancy.[24] In this culture at least, even though women generally endure the actual birth process alone, men have played an active social role in the pregnancy.

In modern Western societies, however, men were often distanced from the pregnancy and excluded from the birth process. The medicalization of pregnancy moved births from the home to the hospital in the early 20th century in the United States, and hospitals would direct fathers into waiting rooms for the majority of the century. Judith Walzer Leavitt, a scholar on birthing practices, takes on the subject of what is happening with the male during birth in her book *Make Room for Daddy*. Men were relegated to special waiting rooms known as "stork clubs," "husbands' rooms," or "fathers' rooms" so they could be near the maternity suites but not able to oversee (or hear) the action in the birthing room. Hospitals would rarely give men very much information about their wives' progress during labor.

Hospitals did sometimes supply journals to men so they could record their thoughts. The journals became the male's connection to the birthing process. They could read the stories of those who had been waiting before them and look for reassurance as they tried to pass time. It was also a way for them to let out their own frustrations with the waiting game.[25] Despite the journals, men were still expected to sit and wait for news of their offsprings' birth in these stork clubs. Hospitals thus institutionalized and medicalized the birth process, and delivered the "results" to fathers only after the birth experience was over.

In the 1950s some doctors who believed in more natural approaches to labor began to include men in the birthing process. An English physician, Dr. Grantly Dick-Read, thought labor pain was brought on by tension. He proposed a natural childbirth, where women would be more relaxed by having the husband with her in the labor room.[26] French physician Fernand Lamaze also thought the father was important in helping the women do breathing exercises to manage pain during labor. In 1965, American doctor Robert A. Bradley also found that having a spouse present could help the mother and encouraged men to join their wives in the labor room to act as their coach.[27]

The feminist movement played a role here too. Feminism asserted that women could only be "free" if men and women were equal; so men had to get involved in places where only women were before. Unlike the imaginary male involved in stories and films of male pregnancies, these new medical and feminist theories encouraged men to become involved in what was before thought to be solely a woman's sphere. Feminists further believed that if men and women could both be a part of the pregnancy and delivery process, men could share a connection to the baby earlier, and in the future, perhaps women would not be "relegated" to being a primary caretaker once the baby was born.

Although men became more accepted in the delivery room, they still faced the problem of what to do once there. Doctors and nurses worked to help deliver the baby and the role of moms was clear, but what was expected of dads? Many men began to describe themselves as "coaches," connoting someone who oversees the process and is responsible for the ultimate "win" (one does not even want to think about the alternative to winning). As coaches, men stood on the sidelines and encouraged women on to the finish line. As the popularity of this concept grew, classes sprung up to teach men how to become successful coaches. Coaches though, are not actual players but leaders or supervisors of a team. Although feminists thought that having men in the delivery room could help to break down gender roles and boundaries, the idea of the father as "coach" may actually encourage a patriarchic system. Instead of a room full of women helping each other through the experience, we now have the doctor (typically during this point in time a male) and another authority figure, now the husband, telling the woman what to do. Despite this, women were relieved to have a friendly presence in the room.

On the other hand, doctors were not necessarily thrilled with the men, now trained to act as coaches, attending the birth. Fathers begin to file lawsuits that claim they had witnessed something going wrong during a birth. One case, *Justus v. Atchison,* involved two sets of parents who were not simply suing for "wrongful" death of their infants but also for pain and suffering of the husbands while they were witnessing the birth.[28] The judge ruled that the men needed to expect some unpleasant experiences while watching the birth. Men were now faced with a dilemma: they wanted to be there for their wives but they did not want to actually witness the uglier side of birth. Medical technology may provide an answer to this problem as it helps to shift men's role in the delivery room.

In August 2006, a husband and wife appeared on the CBS *Early Morning Show* for a video he had taken of his wife's growing pregnant belly and posted on YouTube, which was ranked as the website's top video that week. The husband had used software to speed up the process he had taken of posing his wife each day in front of the same white background so you get to see her belly growing. The video does not sound all that exciting but set to music it shows a beautiful transformation that seemed to capture the public mind. More importantly, the video demonstrates how far men have come in their engagement with the pregnancy and birth process and their use of video for this involvement.

Long before fathers donned video cameras to both preserve the event of the delivery and mediate their own experience, Stan Brakhage, an experimental filmmaker, became known as the father of the birth film. In 1958, he began to film his own children's births. At this point, the birth film was still relegated to the world of an experimental filmmaker—the same man who took the wings of moths and pressed them between two pieces of film and projected them was now filming a birth. To Brakhage, a birth was a beautiful experience and he tried to display it in his film. The feminist and sexual revolutions also occurring at this time were his background. In exposing birth he tried to reveal what was a private and secret experience to a wider audience. He tried to counter the idea of birth as a hidden event and that viewing a birth would not be considered part of an everyday experience.[29] In fact, his wife needed to have the births at home to even provide him with the opportunity to both experience and film them. The film enabled Brakhage to distribute the experience to the public. But since it was an experimental and abstract film, the majority of the public did not see his birth experience.

It was the invention of the camcorder in the 1980s that allowed everyday people to have access to the technology and to start filming births. The video camera was also responsible for helping men find a role in the birth process. They could be there for the birth and the safe confines of a camera could mediate the experience for them. Unlike the birth film of Brakhage, these filmed births were not about birth as art but were simply meant to document the individual experience. The practice of filming a birth has paralleled the fact that it has now become more common for fathers and even other family members to attend a birth. The birth has even become an experience to share with others later in their living rooms, again, through the safe confines of a mediated experience. More people therefore have had the chance to witness and document a birth, even though the opportunity to view videotaped births is generally limited to close family and friends and, more often, simply for the couple themselves (and possibly the children) to view. Men have found a new place for themselves in the delivery room—behind the camera producing a document of the delivery just as the mother produces the baby itself.

But now the birth film has reached a new stage since it is not created simply for men to share with their closest family and friends but also to post on

YouTube for anyone to see. A quick search of YouTube offers an array of different birth videos. And YouTube itself has been pretty liberal regarding the amount of nudity allowed to be depicted in this domain, illustrating how birth may be reaching a phase where it is no longer considered secret and private but considered natural and appropriate to be viewed. This development also allows parents to distribute the filming of a birth to a wide audience.

Mediated technology is encouraging a historical reversal of men's involvement in pregnancy. It used to be that men were passive consumers of pregnancy. They could only experience it through the mother. But now they can construct their own narratives of the pregnancy. In some ways, this technology can bring men closer to the pregnancy as they document the physical progress of the wife as her belly grows. Or, the technology can keep the men busy during the birth with their new jobs. Lance Armstrong "twittered" his newest child's birth, the latest version of a man using technology to spread the news fast.

However, in the same way that the technology may bring men closer to the pregnancy, it can also distance them. One woman shared with me that when her husband was filming her ultrasound, she thought he was not really experiencing the present or the moment with her. Perhaps, men are losing out by witnessing these moments secondhand, or perhaps they are more comfortable in this role instead of watching firsthand a woman they love in pain or watching the exposure of the uglier secrets of birth.

This Is My Labor

Men that have never before been in a position to have children are now also able to experience pregnancy and childbirth in new ways, thanks to new technology. Gay men are increasingly becoming involved in the surrogate and adoption market. The mediated technology of pregnancy along with the social consumption surrounding pregnancy allows them to have an involvement with the pregnancies of birth mothers. The Pop Luck Club is an organization of gay dads in Los Angeles. Interviews with members of this club illustrate gay men who were able to experience pregnancies in their own way.

Those couples who experience adoptions and those involved with surrogacy become involved with the pregnancies at different points. Parents involved in surrogacy generally have a stronger sense of ownership over a fetus but both adoptive parents and surrogate parents seem to experience a pregnancy equally, just at different points in the process. Getting pregnant is also a complicated ritual for gay fathers. They have to decide which path to head down to create the child. This is something that 30 years ago would have been considered complicated but these days, there are plenty of heterosexual couples who are facing difficulties becoming pregnant; so having a process to get a baby seems pretty normal. In fact, while these men sometimes have special agencies focused on them as a consumer group, they often share the same infertility office space with heterosexual couples trying to become pregnant.

Both potential adoptive and potential surrogate couples are in a position of choosing the right woman to help them achieve the process of creating a child. One adoptive couple describes putting together "a loving daddy's book" but none of the men I spoke with describe any type of problem finding a woman to carry their child or give their baby up for adoption. One man, Scott, says picking out the egg donor for his eventual twins "was like shopping on Amazon for the potential biological mother of your child."

The surrogate couples often purposely hire a separate egg donor and surrogate so as to separate the biological and gestational ties to the pregnancy. Technology thus allows the baby to become the biological child of at least one of the men and to also distance the woman carrying the baby from the pregnancy. The result is a woman who is a womb donor but does not have any biological ties to the child. In place of the woman, these men take over the pregnancy experience in a vicarious way. They become involved from the very beginning of the process since they need to donate sperm. And when the pregnancy is successful, they are immediately part of the experience. In fact for some, the pregnancy test stick is the first moment of connecting with their potential baby. The pregnancy test becomes the time when the men embrace and feel involved with the pregnancy. One man, Ru, remembers that moment in which the pregnancy stick came up positive. His surrogate had become pregnant the first time but it had resulted in a miscarriage. Ru experienced the loss immensely and says he was supported by his friends but one can see how his was a unique experience. When the surrogate got pregnant again, she shared his enthusiasm and took three different kinds of pregnancy tests so that she could text them to his cell phone. He still keeps it there as a reminder. The technology functions as a permanent visual reminder of a change in hormones indicating pregnancy, allowing a father to share the conception experience with his surrogate.

The ultrasound is another technology that allows both the surrogate and adoptive dads to experience the pregnancy and meet their baby for the first time. One man, a judge named David, describes the moment when he found out that his baby was a girl. "I thought for sure we were having a boy so when we found out it was a girl you could hear a pin drop—there was dead silence. When we walked out to the parking lot the surrogate said I'm sorry as though it was her fault." He later describes his overwhelming joy in his daughter and how this joy exceeded all of their expectations. For Ru, the ultrasounds were "surreal." He was expecting triplets and his surrogate actually fell asleep during the ultrasound because it was taking a long time to see each baby. He was left alone to experience the ultrasound and view his babies.

There are still moments, though, when fathers of adopted and surrogate children are reminded that they have someone else carrying their baby. This emotion seems most felt by the adoptive fathers, since they become involved in the pregnancy later in the process than the surrogate fathers, and also do not have any biological connection to the child. One man, Matt, describes how he and his partner bonded with their adoptive children's birth mothers (they adopted two different children from two separate mothers). But throughout the process, they kept feeling a need to please the mothers and treat them well. They described two reasons for this need. First, they did not want the woman to change her mind about giving up her child. But they also wanted to be able to later to look their children in the eyes and be able to say that they did all they could for their mothers. As a result, Matt and his partner found themselves putting these women up in housing and making sure to satisfy their cravings and other comforts.

Matt's first experience with an adoptive mother went pretty smoothly but when they adopted their second child they found the experience a bit more strenuous. The adoptive mother required a longer period of care and she was more emotionally and financially needy. After a particularly difficult week, a friend gave him a piece of advice. She told him "You are not going through the physical manifestations. This is the part that you have to play. Suck it up. This is your labor." That phrase became his mantra and he would say to himself "this is your labor" anytime he was feeling overstressed by the experience.

While most of the men describe warm relationships with their surrogates (who they often keep in touch with), they still describe constraints in not being able to control all aspects of the pregnancy. There is a lot of advance discussion about how the surrogate will take care of her body, but the men still worry. Another father, Ben, describes how he wanted to make sure that his surrogate ate enough meat, protein, and leafy greens, since such nutrients are important to a growing fetus. He says, "It very much felt like our pregnancy. Obviously not physically but we were extremely invested and extremely involved."

Ru had to negotiate with his surrogate about the fact that she was carrying triplets. She had agreed before becoming pregnant to reduce the pregnancies, but once pregnant, she felt strongly that she wanted to carry all three. He was left facing conflicting medical advice from doctors who wanted him to reduce and her desire (and his too) to have all three babies. Ultimately, she did end up carrying all three. Matt describes an emotional ultrasound moment: "We were in with this woman that we didn't really know and she's baring it all emotionally and physically. Her stomach was exposed and they were rubbing the gel and putting the sensors around. And it was a surreal moment. We saw the baby and you could see facial features."

Because much of pregnancy has become a sociological experience as much as a biological one, these men are able to experience other rituals that used to be exclusive to the pregnant women. Scott and Dave created their own ritual out of reading their favorite pregnancy book, which was a daily account of what was happening in their surrogate mother's womb. Each night, they would get into bed and read the book together. "We kept a pregnancy journal. We would see her once a month, sometimes a couple of weeks but when we're in bed, we can't feel the stomach (even though she let us do that during her visit)." The book made them feel "present." Although they couldn't be present with their surrogate mother all the time, they found a way to use this book as a way in. Another ritual that all of these couples have done is to enlist family help for the babies' first weeks. They start registering. They also have had elaborate baby showers, given by family and friends, often with alcohol (no need for abstaining) to celebrate the upcoming birth. Sometimes the woman carrying the child is a part of these events, but more often these social components of the pregnancy are the domain of the men.

The experience of these men is unique. They find themselves in infertility clinics but their inability to conceive is not a medical problem but a biological one. New technologies, though, have allowed them an opportunity to partially erase previous biological barriers, and also the opportunity to become involved earlier in the process. Physically, these men still need a woman to carry a baby, but while her womb may be for

"for rent" (or through adoption), the child is all theirs. And they do not have to wait until the baby is born to become involved and experience the pregnancy.

Dad as Commodity

The involvement of the dad in pregnancy is moving earlier in the process. Dads have always had some sort of role in pregnancy. Certainly, their main job was to take care of the mom-to-be in providing food and security. In more modern times, a popular dad role was to build the crib and other toys and products that the baby would need. But the role of the dad-to-be was clearly a secondary role; his job was to support the pregnant mom. But now, the dad-to-be is emerging as a new official position. He is being recognized as playing an important role during this period and having to make his own adjustments. The dad is moving from playing a backseat role in the pregnancy to being recognized as one of the key players.

In the United States, prior to the mid-20th century there were formal ways to become involved in pregnancy but a role was just emerging for the dad in the birth process. Although hospitals often shunned men from being a presence at the actual birth, by the 1970s it began to be recognized that men could serve a role in supporting their wives in pregnancy and childbirth. Classes (such as instruction in the Bradley and Lamaze methods) began to pop up that would prepare men for the birth and the role of labor assistant for the mother. However, these classes did not start until the end of the pregnancy and positioned the dad-to-be as serving the main role of supporting the mom during the actual delivery. Before that, there just was not much to do and the focus of these classes was on the pregnant woman. But now, many dads are becoming part of a movement for equal/shared parenting. In the book, *The Daddy Shift*, Jeremy Adam Smith describes his experiences as a stay-at-home dad while tracing the history and social and political consequences of the trend for more dads to become involved. Ultimately, it is becoming more socially acceptable for dads to become active parents in raising their children.[30] So, why would they want to wait until their babies are already born?

These days, new classes have emerged that are just for dads-to-be, and these classes are happening earlier in the process. On Scott Baio's reality program, we see him attending these dad support group classes during his wife's pregnancy. These classes focus on the feelings of the dad-to-be and his role in pregnancy and childbirth. The starting point of involvement of dads has just gotten earlier. It is now recognized that dads-to-be are at an important juncture and at a time in their lives that is unique for them.

Scientific research is beginning to reflect this with new studies focusing on the dads-to-be. In her book, *The Mommy Brain*, author Louann Brizendine cites research indicating hormonal changes not just in expectant mothers but also for fathers-to-be. Their testosterone levels change in that they have increase in prolactine, a nurturing hormone.[31] Expecting dads no longer need to make fun of their unexpected sympathy weight gain or mood swings—they may be entitled to it. New studies are beginning to examine the mental health of new dads. A study of first-time fathers found that pregnancy is a stressful period of time for men as well as women. Specifically, men are not prepared for how the pregnancy will affect their lives, in particular, their sex lives.[32] The results of this study may seem obvious to any mom-to-be but the significance here is that it is becoming more commonplace now for researchers to turn their attention to examine this unique time in the lives of fathers-to-be.

Armin Brott, the author of numerous books on the experience of pregnancy and parenting from the dad's perspective recognized a void here and has filled it with bestsellers like *The Expectant Father, The New Father,* and *Fathering Your Toddler.* He also has a website and information marketing to this specific audience of dads-to-be. He even does personal coaching for dads or dads-to-be. In other words, he has created a market for giving advice to a group of people who were ignored before. When I interviewed Brott, he talks about the time when he was a new dad and "there were no resources out there—no classes and groups" and "the pregnancy magazines were women's magazines." He worked with a publisher who had found him based on an article he had written about his experiences as one of the only male caregivers on the playground. He knew that he had found his audience: men who wanted to be more involved in pregnancy and birth but needed the appropriate information to become involved. He helped them by not only telling the men to go to the doctor with their wives but by also giving them questions to ask the doctor during the visit.

Brott was not the first one to think of the ways to explore men's role in pregnancy, but the products and services that came before him thought that what men really needed was simply better ways to understand the perspective of the mom-to-be. One such product is the "empathy belly," which enables men to experience pregnancy vicariously—they could put on the empathy belly and be temporarily pregnant. Developed in 1989 by Linda Ware, and manufactured by a company called Birthway, Inc., the product was composed of water and lead weights and even allowed the wearer to experience symptoms ranging from shortness of breath, extra weight, and incontinence (through another bag of water positioned over the bladder).[33] Its main uses was to serve the men trying to empathize with their wives (hence the name), as well as teenagers to give them a fearful taste of what it was like to be pregnant. The belly is positioned as a tool to show just how difficult it is to be pregnant. Men who used it were really treated in the same way as the teenager—you should be lucky you are not pregnant because now you realize that it is very difficult. For the teens it was a warning against getting pregnant and for men it was an admonition to take care of your wife since she is so uncomfortable. Products like these were created with the idea of having men experience the same sensory experience as women. Men could not have a sensory experience with the pregnancy, so products like these were created for men to have their own experience.

But now, marketers have figured out that men want their own sympathy. Take, for example, these shirts sold at Café Press. "Be Nice to Me, The Queen is Pregnant" one reads. Another reads, "You Don't Scare Me, My Wife Is pregnant." Other captions like "He Shoots, He Scores" and "See? My Boys Don't Need to Stop and Ask Directions" allows a man to brag about his ability to impregnate his wife. These shirts encourage the man to glorify his role in the pregnancy. But dads-to-be still have not lost their role of supporting the moms-to-be. The "push present" has become a more commonplace item to appear post-birth. Women expect some type of present (usually in the form of jewelry) to reward them for pushing the baby out. The job of the dad-to-be then is to shop for this token and to reward the wife for the baby they have just had.

Moreover, baby showers, once the domain of just women, have started to become coed. These days, men sometimes have their own baby showers. On the reality program *Tori & Dean,* Tori has her baby shower but simultaneously, Dean's friends meet him for a male version of a baby shower. Today, many men do not want to be left out of the baby shower, or even registering for the products for the baby prior to the baby shower. A quick search online even finds activities and games to involve the dad in the shower. A market is quickly emerging for men but it is a challenging market. Men want to become involved but many resist the femininity attached to the traditional baby shower or baby products. Marketers have to find products that can appear to be more gender neutral.

Dave Campanaro, the Director of Communications for the Brooklyn Cyclones organized an entire group of activities for pregnant woman called "Bellies and Baseball" to encourage pregnant women to come to the baseball game. The event appealed to the dads-to-be as other events were focused specifically for them. One game was called "Water-Break," where the expectant fathers would compete in a race with water balloons on their bodies. In another one, called "Trimester Tricycles," expectant fathers competed in a bike race between innings.

What was once an exclusive domain for women has now opened up to fathers. In many ways, this has been a great boon for couples. They are able to experience the excitement of waiting for the birth, bond earlier with their babies, and help and support each other in new and more effective ways. There are new studies and groups to attend to their needs. At the same time, the men have become a new group for marketers to find and sell to. There is certainly a lot men can do while women are pregnant and it is true that men may require a lot more support at this time in their lives, but in the future we will have to debate which of these services help fathers participate significantly in the pregnancy process and those which serve only the needs of marketers.

Conclusions

Pregnancy has shifted from simply a medical experience to a social one as well. Because of this, pregnancy is no longer the domain only of the female body and of the woman. For some feminists in the 1970s, this was the dream—for women to be liberated from pregnancy so that men could finally experience their "fair share" of the work around childbirth and child care. However, this utopian vision has not been reached exactly according to plan. Instead of women free of the burden of pregnancy, men are simply becoming another group involved with and a part of the pregnancy.

Different types of technology have played a strong role in allowing dads to be engaged. Technology like the pregnancy test, ultrasounds, and stethoscopes that pregnant couples can buy to listen to their babies, all play a role in serving as media that can help the prospective fathers bond with their growing babies in their wives' bellies.

Other media technology has shifted fathers from their role as consumers of pregnancies (through their wives) to producers of the pregnancy. Blogs and twitter allow dads to track the progress of their wives and to chronicle their emotions and feelings as the pregnancy progresses. Video cameras allow dads to record the process and the birth and to serve in this important role as documenter for the pregnancy.

At some point, women have become so peripherally involved in pregnancy that it is possible for another group, like gay men, who have no physical connection to the pregnancy (except perhaps the initial donated sperm) to be able to experience the pregnancy. As women have gained power in the public sphere, they have lost their exclusive domain of pregnancy and childbearing. It is no longer an intimate experience that only women can understand because the entire experience of pregnancy itself has become externalized so that parts of it can be experienced by everyone.

Some may see this as a societal improvement. There may be a breakdown of gender lines and we now have the idea that childbearing (and consequently child-rearing) can also rest with men. Conceptions of masculinity may change as men start to experience a domain that used to be entirely feminized. But this is not so likely to happen now that businesses have seen the potential for a new market. Rather than integrate men into the pregnancy, they would rather create a pregnant experience just for the men—so that they can retain their female market and have a new one as well. So, the feminist dream of males shouldering their burden of the pregnancy is not likely to come true. Instead, there will be more than one type of pregnancy experience, tailored for each sex in society.

Chapter 6

The Pregnancy Industrial Complex

"Just because you're in the hospital and about to have your uterus slashed open, doesn't mean you can't be fashionable."—Tori Spelling, wearing a designer birthing gown that she brought to the hospital, as she was about to give birth via C-section in *Tori & Dean*, season 3. When my mother went to the hospital to have me, she did have a suitcase, but it did not have much inside. She packed some clothes for herself and not knowing if I would be a boy or girl, a few unisex-colored onesies for me. My father remembered his camera, though he could not snap pictures of my arrival since he was not allowed in the delivery room. These days, hospital stays are shorter than ever for most pregnant women, but their suitcases have become full of "necessary" items. The authors of the bestselling pregnancy advice book *What to Expect When You're Expecting* advise to bring the following:[1]

- Their book
- Your birthing plan
- Watch or clock
- Radio or CD player
- Camera, tape recorder, video recorder
- Entertainment (cards, puzzles, etc.)
- Favorite lotions or oils
- Tennis ball or rolling pin
- Your own pillow
- Lollipops or candy
- Toothbrush
- Heavy socks
- Comfortable slippers
- Hairbrush
- Food for your coach
- Bottle of champagne

Some of these items seem sensible; certainly, I can't imagine staying overnight anywhere without a toothbrush, though my hospital actually provided this "luxury" item. The entertainment items, however, seemed puzzling to my mom, who thought waiting for and having her baby was entertaining enough. Other lists remind women to take their iPods and BlackBerries, gifts for older siblings (my mother thought her gift to me was my little sister), and specially designed delivery and nursing gowns so that women do not have to feel like a patient when in the hospital.

When I was born, pregnancy and birth were not separate experiences, but merely the means to a baby. Birth was understood as a medical condition to be experienced in the hospital, and pregnant women were patients. Today, boredom seems to be a disease to cure during birth. A series of consumer experiences replace the community-centered rituals of the past. Pregnancy and birth are two distinct periods that have become fashionable and glamorized by celebrities, promoted and commoditized by companies with a product to sell, and then embraced by moms-to-be as a chance to enjoy and relish this time of their lives.

Hide and Seek

Most people credit Lucille Ball with having the first television baby. In fact, the first American television actress to become pregnant while starring on television was Mary Kay, the star of *Mary Kay and Johnny Stearns,* a fictional program about a couple living in New York City that aired during 1947–1950. Because Mary Kay and Johnny played a television version of themselves, when Mary Kay became pregnant, the couple wrote their pregnancy into the show. The real Mary Kay gave birth just a half hour before her television delivery aired.[2] But, despite Mary Kay's position as the first official television birth, it is with good reason that Lucille Ball gets all the credit.

Yes, more people were watching television in the early 1950s, and *I Love Lucy* consistently ranked among the top programs at the time. However, Ball's televised birth went beyond Mary Kay to become the first televised birth that was also a media event. Not coincidentally, Ball was scheduled for a C-section the same day that her television baby was born. The ratings for the fictional birth drew close to 44 million viewers.[3] While Mary Kay was the first to merge her birth experience with her character, Ball had what we now call a celebrity birth.

Despite this extensive coverage, magazine covers focused not on Ball's pregnancy itself, but on the expectation of her baby's arrival. More than a euphemism for the forbidden word pregnancy, "expecting" reveals the

perspective of this time: pregnancy was little more than a period of anticipation, a necessary inconvenience that nature required in order to become
transformed into the venerable role of mother.

Pregnancy and birth have since moved out of the secluded delivery
room. We no longer wait until the day the baby comes to start talking,
wondering, and speculating about it. Tabloids have begun to out pregnant
celebrities. Fans search for belly bumps. From its ubiquitous perch on the
checkout line at the supermarket, *People* magazine each week shows off
another pregnant star. This was not always the case. If you compare current issues of the magazine with issues from its debut year in 1974, you will
find a society where pregnancy was hidden and not spoken about publicly.

In the 1970s, *People* rarely discussed pregnancy, and when it did, it was
often as a secondary or minor part of a story. For example, a story on Hay-
ley Mills reported that she gave birth to a son, Crispian, 16 months earlier.
The article, titled "Mother Mill," used Crispian's birth to promote Mill's
starring role in *The Family Way,* but remarkably avoided many details
about Mill's own pregnancy.[4] Celebrating the birth of Lyndon and Lady
Bird Johnson's grandchild, *People* published a photo of their daughter Luci
leaving the hospital with her new baby. The picture artfully frames Luci
waist-up, so as to avoid showing her postpartum body.[5]

On the rare occasions when *People* featured pregnant celebrities within
their pages, accompanying photographs either hid or detracted from the
pregnancy. For example, a story announced that Rick Nelson and his wife
Kristin were expecting another baby. The caption under the photo reads,
"While the pregnant Kristin relaxes with a book, Rick tries out one of his
new songs at the piano."[6] The caption describing Kristin as pregnant was
necessary, one may argue, because the picture artfully positioned Kristin's
pregnant belly out of frame. Despite the celebration of women's liberation
and sexual freedom, pregnancy was rarely shown and hardly mentioned
in part because of a lingering sensitivity toward discussing sex in public.
Pregnancy was a too in-your-face reminder of where babies come from.

When stories in *People* did focus on pregnancy, they often approached
the topic from a medical perspective. In a column titled "Medics," a doctor advises on the merits of the novel and unorthodox practice of a home
birth. Because of the prevailing attitude of the day of pregnancy as a medical condition, the magazine misses any trace of irony when it addresses
home birth, a nonmedical approach to pregnancy, within a medical column.[7] Even medical depictions employ a modest tone. Pictures of doctors examining women have their shirts cover their bellies.[8] Another story,
about a doctor delivering a baby, shows only a picture of the mother's face.[9]

While the *People* magazine of 1974 did not dwell on pregnancy, it did focus on issues of motherhood and feminism. For instance, a column called "Lookout" (another discontinued column) quoted the rising feminist Sheli Rosenberg: "Equal employment for women is not a fair issue until we come to grips with the problems of motherhood."[10] Stories about celebrity mothers skip over their pregnancies and instead highlight their difficulties trying to balance fame with the social pressure of being a wife and mother. Barbara Walters discusses her effort to not allow her career to interfere with motherhood, worrying that she would miss her daughter (Jackie, aged six) growing up. Jane Withers, the star of *Josephine the Plumber,* has come back to work after taking time off to become a wife and mother of five. The caption under her photo reassures readers: "Still putting her family first despite her new career."[11] During this period, the magazine concentrated on women's attempts to balance family and career, rather than the process of creating that family.

Contrast this to the *People* magazine of today, which often displays pregnant women prominently on its cover. Headlines scream slogans like, "She's Having My Babies," promoting a story about Joan Lunden's relationship with her surrogate, and "Baby Boom," teasing an issue that celebrates the pregnancies of Gwyneth Paltrow and Geena Davis. A flattering photo of Reese Witherspoon on the cover is accompanied by the caption, "Baby on the Way?" The related story advances rumors that Witherspoon is pregnant with her second child, before she has made her pregnancy public.

Instead of pretending that the act of conception has nothing to do with pregnancy, today celebrities talk openly about sex. Angelina Jolie, one of the most-watched pregnant celebrities, discussed having sex while pregnant. "It's *great* for the sex-life," she freely offers. "It just makes you a lot more creative so you have fun and as a woman, you're just so round and full."[12] Rather than skipping over the birth process when discussing his son's birth, Matthew McConaughey described the scene in detail to *OK* magazine, saying: "Having a baby is a bloody, pukey, sweaty, primeval thing."[13] *People* has replaced its medical column with "Expecting," a column that details the latest celebrity pregnancy. And, if the magazine is not enough, readers can go the *People*'s celebrity baby blog, where they can track pregnant celebrities and see glimpses of them with their children. Pregnancy, once hidden by publishers, has become a regular component of celebrity publicity.

But this shift in how magazines cover pregnancy influences how readers perceive pregnancy and motherhood. Magazines have moved from covering what is going on inside the belly as a medical issue to simply following the belly itself. Feminism and the politics of pregnancy have given way to personal issues. Pregnant women are much more visible in these pages, but only when they serve to glorify pregnancy and motherhood. Susan Douglas and Meredith Michaels label this phenomenon the "New Momism." They assert that stories in these magazines encourage a society that allows women to feel fulfilled only when they have children and become completely involved in their lives.[14] A prime example is *US Weekly*'s issue called "Hot Mamas!" that explains "Why Hollywood's sexy young screen queens want babies now."

For many celebrities, their pregnancy offers a chance to connect with fans. Unlike a celebrity wedding, pregnancy is a relatable moment that physically transforms the body. Celebrities gain weight and suffer the same side effects as any other pregnant woman, making them seem more human. However, in the retouched world of celebrity news, pregnant celebs seem to "do" pregnancy better than anyone else. The glorification of celebrity pregnancy paints a world where celebrities simply revel in their newfound, worry-free motherhood.

In fact, many celebrities struggle with the press in deciding when to announce their pregnancies to the public. Jennifer Lopez and Marc Anthony tried to control their announcement by refusing to confirm her pregnancy despite endless media speculation, and her growing belly. Finally, Lopez declared she was pregnant during one of her concerts. A fan posted the announcement on YouTube, but few were surprised.

Bethenny Frankel, a star of the reality programs *The Real Housewives of New York City* and *Bethenny Getting Married*, took another approach. When celebrity blogger Perez Hilton spread rumors of her pregnancy, she regained control by granting an interview with *People* magazine. In the interview, she confirmed her pregnancy but as she was less than three months along, she felt a formal announcement was premature.

Gisele Bundchen, a supermodel and wife of football player Tom Brady, created a stir in the blogosphere when she posed in a trench coat for London Fog. The company had airbrushed her belly bump out of the photograph, citing privacy concerns, as the couple had not yet announced the pregnancy. Despite this explanation, bloggers were upset that the company and Gisele were not relishing and showing off her bump. Rather than disappearing from public view, celebrities can now get a "digital abortion," wiping clean any traces of pregnancy in images and wresting control of the pregnancy back from the fans.

Celebrities face pregnancy scrutiny even before they become pregnant. Fans and the tabloid press have replaced the nagging mother in pressuring celebrities to conceive. They look for baby bumps, question when celebrity couples will have a child and why they have not already started. Even when babies do come, they speculate on how the pregnancy happened. Multiple births are immediately cast with suspicion as the tabloids speculate whether the celebrities used fertility treatments to facilitate the pregnancy. Some tabloids accused Angelina and Brad of using in vitro fertilization to produce twins to grow their large family even faster.

The pregnancy and birth of hip-hop star Beyoncé is a perfect illustration of the challenges facing celebrities both trying to promote and guard their pregnancies. She publicly announced her pregnancy by rubbing her protruding belly during the MTV Video Music Awards.[15] During her pregnancy, Beyoncé was proud to show. To preserve her privacy during her birth at a Manhattan hospital, she arranged for her own private security team. Controversy ensued when several nonfamous couples complained, and the news media picked up on the story, about how they were restricted access from their own children while security took over the floor, and blocked hospital security cameras. Apparently, the security staff wore special badges labeled "special event," which further insulted those "regular new moms" who also thought of their births as special.[16] Beyoncé, of course, faced a real conflict with a public that had been following her pregnancy and was now reaching a moment that she wanted to retain for herself, for both privacy and security reasons.

Media coverage of celebrity pregnancy has come full circle. In the past, when a woman became pregnant, she retreated from public view. Now, celebrities are forced to do a dance with the press over whether to reveal or conceal their pregnancies. Technology has made it harder to make these decisions. Digital cameras, the 24-hour news cycle, and the growth of websites and blogs have all created an environment in which celebrities are constantly watched. While the media of the past simply ignored pregnancy, today the celebrities are in a battle to retain control of when their pregnancy becomes public.

Maternity Clothing

A reader's letter in *People* magazine in 2003 expressed shock over the appearance of Kate Hudson baring her belly. The reader lamented, "There is nothing more lovely than a pregnant woman, especially one who carries herself with grace and dignity. . . . Kate Hudson, by baring her belly, disgraces herself and other expectant mothers. Kate, look in the mirror."[17] Clearly, not everyone feels that the pregnant body is something to show off. Yet these days, not only do pregnant women avoid the previous century's practice of hiding in their houses while pregnant, they also wear clothes that accentuate their pregnancy. Instead of hiding the womb, it is highlighted by contemporary maternity fashion.

From the early 17th through the 20th centuries, pregnant women tended to cover and hide any evidence of the fetus growing inside them. Many did so out of concern for the fetus, as doctors told women that loose clothes were better for the baby. They cautioned expectant women that tight-fitting clothes could impact "expansion of the womb, and in consequence, of the foetus [sic]."[18] These concerns were not completely unfounded, as many women still wore corsets until the mid-19th century. Even after medically dangerous corsets fell out of style, an advice book for pregnant women published in 1904 warned, "A lady who is pregnant ought on no account to wear tight dresses, as the child should have plenty of room." It continues: "Let the clothes be adapted to the gradual development both of the belly and the breasts. She must, whatever she may usually do, wear her stays loose."[19]

Examining these advice books reveals that women in the 19th century had to be persuaded to wear loose clothing not because they wanted to show off their bellies, but because they did not want to indicate in public that they were pregnant at all. "Great errors in dress are sometimes committed by young women when they become pregnant for the first time," one book cautioned. "They do not accommodate their dress to their new situation, desirous (from mistaken feelings of delicacy) to conceal the fact from observations as long as possible."[20] Maternity clothing was varied by class. Upper class women could wear dressing gowns in private but had to find more formal clothing for public appearances. A popular style in 1851 was the jacket-style bodice. Part of its appeal was that it buttoned in the front and was able to hide the waistline. This new dress served two purposes: it communicated a change in the woman's expecting status while reducing the visibility of the pregnancy, which was still not considered acceptable at the time.[21] Of course, most women did not have the means to purchase this specialized clothing, as mass-marketed maternity dresses did not yet exist, so they were forced to alter their existing clothing.[22]

By the 20th century, advice books shifted the discussion about maternity clothing from its medical benefits to its emotional appeal. A nurse writing in 1937 recommends that women focus on how the clothing may make them feel:

Remembering that it is important for you to keep up the diversions and amusements that you enjoy, it is worthwhile to have your clothes as pretty and becoming as possible, for you are much more likely to go about and mingle with your friends if you feel that you are becomingly and well dressed. At the same time your clothes should be so made that their weight will hang from the shoulders instead of from the waistband.[23]

The first specifically designed maternity clothes appear during this period. In 1904, a dressmaker named Lena Bryant created an accordion pleat dress that allowed for expansion. An advertisement promised that the dress allowed women to be able to live "a normal lifestyle while pregnant."[24] Maternity clothes as a trend had arrived, but they were still designed to hide and minimize the pregnancy. The Lena Bryant maternity line became so popular that the designer followed it with an entire brand of clothing called Lane Bryant. This brand is well known today for providing clothing for "bigger-sized" women. Lena Bryant's specialty as a designer was hiding both the shapes of obesity and pregnancy. For most of the 20th century, maternity clothing is perceived in this way, as a way to hide the "fatness" of pregnancy.

By the end of the 20th century, designers left behind shapeless, oversized designs for more fitted maternity clothing. In the 1990s, designer Liz Lange introduced a fitted maternity line that created such a following that the fashion-conscious stores Target and Nike requested that Lange produce custom lines for their pregnant customers. Gap and Old Navy quickly followed suit with their own maternity brands. That these stores have sought to capture the maternity fashion market demonstrates that women no longer hibernate during their pregnancies, unfit for public displays of fashion. Rather, designers have embraced pregnancy as merely another phase in a woman's life. Rather than lose their customers for the better part of a year, stores have created maternity lines so women can keep dressing in their favored styles and brands of clothes throughout their pregnancy.

While maternity clothing has changed to show off instead of hide the pregnant belly, what has not changed is the class difference in maternity choices, often produced by the same manufacturers. These differences can be readily seen within Destination Maternity, where several different maternity brands are housed under one roof. The upscale Pea in the Pod offers exclusive maternity clothing for women with more money to spend, including a line of clothes designed by former Hollywood Bad Girl/ Heiress Nicole Richie. Motherhood Maternity sells less expensive designs for those on a budget. Maternity clothes have become so marketable that fashion icons have begun to create their own lines. Supermodel Heidi

Klum, host of *Project Runway,* has created two new maternity brands to appeal to both markets. One line, called "Lavish," is described as: "A fashionable expression of everything you want to give yourself and to the child growing within you." Klum has called her less expensive line "Loved" and describes it as: "A celebration of style to match the abundance of love all around you and your baby."[25] Rosie Pope created a maternity line, Rose Pop Maternity that includes clothes and accessories. Her line's popularity among the wealthy set propelled her into her own successful television reality program, *Pregnant in Heels,* chronicling her work as a pregnancy concierge.

These descriptions illustrate a shift in the purpose and function of maternity clothes. In the past, women modified their own clothing without concern for fashion, since they were expected to stay out of the public eye. Then, the first maternity fashions allowed upper-class women to appear in public while concealing their condition. Now, maternity lines allow women to express their own fashion sense while exclaiming their joy in their pregnancy by accentuating, rather than hiding, their bellies with glamorous styles. Others have suggested that, since more women are older when they become pregnant, they have already developed a sense of style that they are not ready to give up.[26] With more disposable income and a desire to appear fashionable in public, older women can afford to indulge in designer maternity clothes.

The reach of maternity fashion has extended to unexpected brands. Forever 21, a popular clothing line that targets a youth market has come under fire for developing a youth maternity line.[27] Critics worry that the chain is glamorizing teen pregnancy with their line, while supporters dismiss these concerns by pointing out that older women are purchasing these clothes. The chain has recognized that women today want to continue to dress young and hip, even when pregnant.

In fact, maternity fashions have gone beyond merely clothing the pregnant woman to focusing on the pregnancy itself by announcing, advertising, and advocating for the fetus. A popular shirt sports baby feet on the front accompanied by the phrase, "What's kickin." Other shirts say, "I can grow people," and "My lovely baby bump."[28] These shirts glorify pregnancy and the ability to carry a baby. They may be hip and cool, but imagine what they must read like to women who are infertile and unable to "grow people." In fact, one may wonder if the shirts express relief more than pride, as more women wait until later in life to have children and are facing more fertility problems. The celebration of pregnancy may be more of a celebration of the *ability* to become pregnant.

Maternity fashion sales jumped 28 per cent from 2000 to 2005.[29] While designers have reacted to the desire for women to dress trendy, technological and social changes also have contributed to the popularity of maternity fashions. As the pregnant body is displayed more often, both externally as women remain in public work and leisure spheres throughout their pregnancy and internally via ultrasounds that make the fetus itself visible, society has developed a tolerance, even a desire, to gaze at the pregnant body. Therefore, maternity clothes have expectedly capitalized on these trends for pregnant women. Take, for instance, the pregnant bride.

Today, the purpose of maternity clothes has undergone a reversal. One trend, in particular, that illustrates this shift is the pregnant bride. In the past, when an unmarried women found out she was pregnant, a marriage ceremony was hastily arranged before she "showed." These days, not only do visibly pregnant women plan elaborate wedding ceremonies, but they also can go to specialty shops to have a maternity wedding dress designed for them.[30] One company, TeKay Designs, is an Internet retailer that specializes in wedding dresses and other formal wear for pregnant women. One can simply peruse the choices on their website and order a wedding dress online. MaternityBride.com showcases the Jessica Iverson couture line, which offers several designs for pregnant brides, mostly in white. On an episode of *Bethenny Getting Married*, pregnant Bethenny purposely chose a dress that accentuated her belly because she wanted to "own the bump." From its genesis as a concealer of pregnancy, changes in maternity clothing reflect the social acceptance of the pregnant body and the working pregnant woman.

The Belly Bump

In 1991, people picked up the August issue of *Vanity Fair* to find Demi Moore posing naked on the cover. Beyond the normal shock of seeing a celebrity nude, her visibly pregnant body stirred a debate over the image's appropriateness. Scholars, critics, and the popular press cite this moment as a critical shift in the cultural perception of pregnancy. Suddenly, celebrity pregnancy was transformed from a public announcement to public spectacle. This moment rested on a broad foundation, however. Ultrasound technology developed over the last 20 years had already made it possible to peer into the previously mysterious pregnant belly and changes in the perception of women and the power they wield gave them more control over their own bodies. Previously private parts can now be displayed with pride. It is no wonder that the exposure of the pregnant body would follow.[31] The Demi Moore image has been repeated by many celebrities in succeeding decades. Just to name a few, Britney Spears posed in *Harper's Bazaar* in 2006, Christina Aguilera chose *Marie Claire* for her close-up in 2008, Mariah Carey was seen with her naked belly bump in *Life & Style*, and, recently, Jessica Simpson added her naked belly to the list in 2012 with her appearance on *Elle Magazine.*

Koren Reyes found her niche in what to her seemed an unlikely clientele. She specializes in maternity pictures. Having always been fascinated with the human figure, she left behind a job in finance to begin a career in photography. She describes the pregnant belly as "this beautiful form; I'm very drawn to it." After shooting pregnant models, and advertising her services, clients immediately began to book sittings. Reyes finds photographing pregnant women completely different than another common life event. "It's unlike a wedding, where there is all kinds of background and emotions going on and there is so much stress and this rush, get it, get the shot, did I miss it," she explains. "Pregnancy is a different kind of experience." She schedules no more than one pregnant client per day so that she can make them comfortable and allow them to enjoy the experience. The pictures she takes focuses on the belly. She prefers that women wear open-neckline shirts in grays, whites, and blacks so the focus is on the belly. She also discourages moms-to-be from wearing anything too trendy so that the portrait retains a timeless allure.

Reyes says her clients often feel self-conscious about their figures. "They feel unattractive, but then they see the pictures and you hear them say, 'You made me look beautiful. I had no idea I looked like that'!" As a photographer, Reyes creates an image of them in the language they have become comfortable with: they interpret their beauty within the perspective of the fashion photograph. She offers higher-priced packages for those who want to be treated like a celebrity for a day. "$7,695 for an all-day luxury experience," her website advertises. "Want a glimpse into the professional world of fashion photography?" The allure of the high-end package is not the shot but the shoot. As more celebrities imitate Moore's iconic pose, the celebrity pregnant belly portrait has become another ideal for women to imitate. The photos are glamorized, touched up by publishers to make them look perfect, and Reyes provides that same level of service to her clients. "I'm no purist," she says. Although she offers to provide images without retouching, most of her clients choose to have their portraits airbrushed. Given the choice between preserving an image of their pregnant body and an idealized version of that image, most women choose the idealization.

Although Reyes's clients choose to photograph themselves like a celebrity, they do not usually display those photographs publicly. Reyes says most women place them in areas of their homes where they can control access. One woman hung three large posters of herself in her bathroom. Other women often put them inside a walk-in closet. In a sense, these photographs function like a ritualized shrine. The pregnant belly, long a traditional symbol of fertility and goodness, now has become personalized. Not quite their baby's first picture, these photographs show the mother-to-be as a vessel for that baby's journey and these women can adulate this time in their life even when they are well past it.

Women also revere their pregnant bellies with temporary tattoos and belly casts. Tattoos, traditionally associated with religious and ritualistic observances, today have become more of a hip form of self-expression. The burgeoning pregnant belly provides a new place for that self-expression. As clothes have allowed pregnant bellies more exposure, the tattoos are visible to the public, and they often communicate with them. Phrases like, "This belly rocks," "Kiss me, I'm pregnant," and "Will kick for ice cream" invite a light-hearted attitude toward the belly and what it represents. Like pregnancy, these tattoos are temporary; they can be safely removed at will, disconnecting them from their traditional purpose as a permanent commitment to a group or ritual. It devalues the tattoo of real meaning.

Belly casts serve a different purpose than tattoos. Like the pictures that Reyes shoots, the casts are a physical manifestation of the pregnant belly. Some women cast their belly as a part of a ritual, such as a baby shower. Others use the moment to involve the expectant dad who is needed to physically help with the actual casting. Most women purchase these products to celebrate and commemorate their pregnant bellies, but objectifying the belly opens it up to a more dystopian future.

The pregnant belly is one of the last noncommercialized spaces, but this status is quickly disappearing. Asia Francis and Amber Rainey are two women who auctioned off on eBay the space on their bellies to advertisers. A web hosting company and a casino purchased the right to place their logos on these women, mostly for the publicity value of doing so.[32] These extreme examples illustrate the commoditization of the pregnant belly as it becomes simply another commercial vehicle.

Pregnancy Lifestyle: "Live it, Then Have it"

From the outside, Ten Toes looks like a typical children's boutique. Once inside, however, a large open space greets visitors. The proprietors, Kathy

Lewis and Leslie Potenciano, have opened a unique business that runs largely on word-of-mouth. Their clients, pregnant women and new moms, have found in Ten Toes a resource for information about pregnancy and parenting. The business offers birthing and parenting classes, hard-to-find specialty products, and motherly advice for the modern family all in one space.

Lewis and Potenciano are both licensed physician assistants. While working at a busy hospital, they constantly fielded questions from pregnant women that they triaged. "Today's physician doesn't have the time to sit and go over everything in the *What to Expect when You're Expecting* book," Lewis says. Potenciano agrees: "The biggest reason why this came about was that a lot of the patients that we saw in the hospital were uninformed, not because they didn't want to know but they didn't have a place to go to ask." They soon realized that what women needed was a place to go where knowledgeable people could answer questions about not just the medical aspects of pregnancy, but the entire pregnant lifestyle. Although their clients cross socioeconomic backgrounds, they tend to be well educated and accustomed to seeking out information from reliable sources.

Classes at Ten Toes differ from traditional childbirth classes: they begin early in the pregnancy. "Instead of waiting until the end of the pregnancy, when you don't like sitting through it," Lewis says, "we like to do it in a broad sense throughout the pregnancy." She adds that, when a woman is pregnant, "You have to live it and then have it." They start their classes at 18 weeks, and women learn about not just the birth but also the emotional and biological changes that pregnancy brings.

Although they sell products at their store, that business is secondary and is provided more as a service to their clients. Potenciano says, "A lot of people ask us for our own recommendations, so we thought it would be a good idea to house the things that we recommend." Their focus is nourishing pregnant women and new moms with information. For both of them, it becomes personal. Over time they get to know their clients, and those relationships sometimes survive even after women give birth. Lewis says, "I always say when I'm having another class that I feel like I'm having another baby."

The Ten Toes center is part of a growing movement of people and companies that are contributing to the idea of pregnancy as a lifestyle. Babeland, a national chain, advertises "sex toys for a passionate world." Perhaps not the first business one would associate with pregnancy; this chain is capitalizing on the trend of pregnant women who are following the Angelina Jolie model of retaining their sexuality while pregnant. Every Tuesday

Babeland hosts a Sexy Mom series at its Brooklyn location. "Sex during and after pregnancy" is just one topic in a regular series of seminars designed to appeal to moms or moms-to-be. Once a taboo topic, sexual activity during pregnancy has become acceptable enough to create a new consumer segment for marketers.

Like services that have created markets exclusively for pregnant women, "chick-lit" has segmented into a subcategory known as the belly-bump book. Pregnancy was not always so visible in literature. Prior to the 20th century, childbirth rarely appeared in fiction, and if it did, it was presented from an audience's point of view. Readers were given the perspective of the father, the doctor, or others in attendance, but never the mother's. Moreover, male critics responded with distaste, finding childbirth scenes repugnant. Thus for the most part, accounts of childbirth were found only in women's private writings or in anonymous letters to magazines.[33]

Now though, characters in chick-lit novels are beginning to find themselves pregnant. Some of these books focus on characters struggling to get pregnant, such as Sinead Moriarty's *The Baby Trail*. Others find themselves unexpectedly pregnant. In Erin McCarthy's *The Pregnant Test*, the protagonist deals with pregnancy after losing her boyfriend and business. Many books just glory in the pregnancy itself. Sophie Kinsella's main character in her Shopaholic series, Becky, becomes pregnant in the fifth book, *Shopaholic & Baby*. Becky is addicted to shopping, and she uses her pregnancy as an excuse to buy more products. She struggles to be a "yummy mummy" through her clothes and accessories and she does not let her pregnancy get in the way of consuming. Laura Wolf followed her *Diary of a Mad Bride* with *Diary of a Mad Mom-to-Be*. The checklist-obsessed main character achieves her goal of getting pregnant and then begins a long list of what to do while pregnant, from what to eat to what to buy. The pregnancy becomes another item to check off her list. The pregnancy ritual these books promote is shopping.

Expectant women can now shop at places that have been designed specifically for them. Spas now offer special packages for moms-to-be. New York City boasts the Edamame Maternity Spa, which only takes pregnant woman as its customers.

Celebrities are begging to capitalize on this new market. In 2005, Kim D'Amato, a former model, opened Priti, a spa that specializes in all-natural products. Her inspiration was her own pregnancy, when she sought out an organic beauty routine that would not harm her baby.[34] With expectant mothers uncertain about the effects of products on their fetuses, ecologically friendly products are naturally appealing to them. Former *Punky*

Brewster child actress Soleil Moon Frye owns The Little Seed, a store that offers green alternative products for expectants moms and babies. Her website, www.thelittleseed.com, includes links to green diets for safer pregnancies.

Seeing its untapped potential, established brands are attempting to capture the pregnancy market. Stonyfield Farms, makers of organic yogurt for babies and kids, introduced YoMommy, designed specifically for the expectant mom. A press release from the company promotes the product as, "The first yogurt created to address the specific nutritional needs of pregnant, nursing and new moms, and their growing babies."[35] The popular skin lotion brand Curel launched a new "Life's Stages" line with a special "nurturing comfort moisture cream for pregnancy & motherhood." It boasts that it has been "developed with OB/GYNs to address dry skin issues during pregnancy. This fast-absorbing cream helps your skin withstand the changes of pregnancy by increasing elasticity over 100 per cent, helping to smooth the appearance of stretch marks."[36] Pregnancy is no longer an inconvenient time for a woman to get through; instead, these products offer the chance to retain the normalcy of her lifestyle, including the ability to purchase health and beauty products.

Marketing companies are beginning to emerge that can connect pregnant women with these new products. "Do you speak pregnancy? We do," is the tag line of Julia Beck's firm Forty Weeks. Her company targets expectant and new parents. Beck describes the moment when she realized companies needed a guiding hand to appeal to this particular market: "I was pregnant with my first child, and I suddenly became the target of people's marketing. They spoke to me in a language of pastels, pinks and blues, and ducks and bunnies. It really felt as if I was being marketed to as if I were the fetus inside of me."

Since then, she began building a business that educates companies on the uniqueness of this particular market. "You will never find a consumer at this crossroad where there is affluence and openness," she explains, "A consumer who is that unsure as to what comes next." Beck argues that other markets behave differently. Tweens have clear ideas of what they like and dislike and brides know exactly what they want in a wedding. But, expectant couples have to gear up quickly and are "at the bottom of a learning curve, so information that is received comes with a very open mind." Beck's company works to address these problems for the expectant mom. She connects companies with philanthropy that will help women during pregnancy and new motherhood. When her client, Bravado Designs, wanted to market their breast-feeding bras, she encouraged them to set up a breast-feeding information council for women. Beck sees her business as unique because her approach is to advise companies to understand the pregnant woman as a person and not simply a buyer.

Companies marketing exclusively to pregnant women help to create a pregnant lifestyle. This brings new levels of enjoyment for women, with products that pamper them and give them the pleasure of shopping for their baby-to-be. With this enjoyment, however, comes a new anxiety, as women attempt to negotiate the bombardment of services and offerings. Women are alleviating their confusion by turning to professional guidance.

The Baby Planner

New Yorkers competing to hire a single, childless man that they have never met to become their consultant for baby-to-be purchases may seem absurd. Yet in 2010, *New York Magazine* labeled Jamie Grayson as the "Best Baby Gear Guru."[37] Like the prevalence of bottled water, women now pay for advice they used to get for free. An episode of *Rachael Ray* featured Ellie and Melissa, West Coast baby planners whose motto is "We take the labor out of delivery."[38] The baby planning industry is ready to fill the knowledge void left when women have countless choices but no longer have a village of neighbors to guide them through what was once a communal process.

Mary Oscategui is the founder and CEO of The International Academy of Baby Planners Professional. Having a medical background, she sees herself as a useful resource during an anxious time in a woman's life. Like many of the other women who find themselves in pregnancy and motherhood-related businesses, Oscategui herself was pregnant when she realized the need for her kind of service: "During my pregnancy, I lacked family support. My family was back East and my partner's family was in Hawaii. . . . My midwife connected me with the support that I needed. She found me a doula and an expert. I got such an amazing support system, and I just felt so empowered."

Each pregnancy is different, so she personalizes her services. "I actually do a client intake," Oscategui says. She goes into clients' homes and evaluates them for both physical and psychological needs. "Which areas need the most attention?" she asks. "Is there an emotional need?" Her goal is to offer women a service that she feels is lacking from the medical establishment. She wants to help women who do not have the family support that some other women have. For those who do have support, she wants to be the person who gathers information for them in one place and offers them clear choices. She differentiates herself from baby planners who cater to the luxury market and focus on the consumer aspect of pregnancy. In fact, the expectant moms she caters to are not interested in that type of service: "The product part they enjoyed doing themselves. Most of the time they can't justify paying $150 to just get product advice, especially with all the bloggers out there, and they might ask, 'What credentials do they have to give me this advice'? So, I was realizing, wow, if I really want to cater to a more mainstream market, I really need to do my work and my research." She found that her health and fitness background provided an understanding of the medical options surrounding birth and the need for postpartum support. Oscategui explains, "A lot of women, they felt most vulnerable right after pregnancy." Her services help women during this time.

Oscategui has networked with other baby planners with similar views, creating an association and academy to focus on training baby planners. The organization addresses all kinds of ethical and practical questions. For example, what happens if practitioners and vendors recommended by them do not provide good service? What should be the responsibilities of the baby planner? Which baby planners should be allowed to dispense medical advice? What credentials should a baby planner have? She, like the other planners in her association, is often hired by companies to give lectures and lead discussions for employees who want to understand and navigate the changing pregnancy experience.

These questions raise the issue of what happens when an industry replaces family and friends in providing advice. How should a woman give birth? What is the best way to take care of a woman after birth? Which products are really needed, and which are merely luxuries? In the past, a daughter could simply ignore a mother's bad advice, as experience teaches her other options. But, bad advice from a professional could very well lead to a lawsuit. Furthermore, this burgeoning industry gives advice on subjects about which there is still much debate. In her book *The Outsourced Self*, Arlie Russell Hochschild laments the degree to which we have come to rely on experts in all aspects of our life: "The very ease with which we reach for market services may also prevent us from noticing the remarkable degree to which the market has come to dominate our very ideas about what can or should be for sale or rent, and who should be included in the dramatic cast—buyers, branders, sellers—that we imagine as part of a personal life."[39] These professionals have stepped in to fill a gap left by a postindustrial society, where women, often physically separated from their mothers, do not have a built-in support system. For some women, baby planners provide an invaluable service. However, they run the danger of displacing instinct, and mistakes that are a natural part of the learning process.

Pregnancy Rituals

Moving from a couple to a family has always been a significant transition, marked with religious and cultural rituals. However, publicly announcing and celebrating the pregnancy now has become an essential part of this transition. Baby showers have moved from a casual ritual to a more formal event. In the past, a few female family members and friends may have gotten together to celebrate this important life shift. They were called baby showers, a time when women would initiate the mother-to-be into the world of baby care. Now, baby showers are an opportunity to celebrate with every acquaintance and to accumulate as many products as possible. Today, most women have more than one baby shower: one at their office, one for family and friends, and sometimes even an additional one for those who could not make the first two. In fact, showers are no longer restricted to women. Some coed showers are so large in their guest lists and cost that they have begun to resemble a wedding reception.

Celebrity baby showers provide a view into the most lavish celebrations. Jennifer Lopez had her baby shower on the rooftop of the Gramercy Park Hotel. The guests received gold-encrusted pacifiers.[40] Celebrity moms-to-be are turning their showers into publicity events. Tori Spelling featured her baby shower on her reality television program. Target and Liz Lange hosted a baby shower for Brooke Shields and were able to promote their new line of maternity clothes simultaneously. Fans can even be virtual guests at other celebrity showers. Tyra Banks hosted Jessica Alba's baby shower on her talk show, and the audience for *The View* watched Elizabeth Hasselbeck share her baby shower with a studio audience filled with pregnant women.

The publicity for these celebrity showers usually focuses on expensive and unique designer products for the woman who already has everything. Marketers view these celebrity events as a model for reorienting the baby shower into a consumer opportunity. Websites have sprouted up that offer shower ideas, themes, and merchandise for any woman to plan an elaborate baby shower.[41] If the baby shower of the past was a place to learn from others about how to become a mother, the baby shower of today is about receiving products that will supposedly make the guest of honor a better mother.

The baby shower is only one of several ways people are marking the transition into parenthood today. Even before the traditional baby shower, some couples are now celebrating with a new type of party: the gender-reveal party. Peggy, a mother of two children, told me the story about the public moment when she found out the sex of her baby. When she was pregnant for the first time, she had an ultrasound but her husband was delayed at work and she was really upset because she didn't want to find out the sex of the baby without him. "I just had such a clear image/fantasy of that moment where we'd both be looking at our baby on the screen, all gray and blurry and barely identifiable as human, but Our Baby, and hear "it's a ___!" Luckily, the doctor had an idea. She said she'd write it down and seal it in an envelope, and we could open it together." When she came home, she expected to open the envelope right away but her husband had another idea. He suggested they have a party and open it up then. "I kept the envelope in my desk at home for something like 2 months (!!!), and then we had a party where we invited a bunch of family and friends, and we all found out together that it was a boy." They had so much fun that even though her husband could have been at the ultrasound for their second child, they asked for another envelope and had another party.

When Peggy's first child was born in 2001, the creation of the party happened organically, as part of a desire to be connected to the pregnancy as a couple, but these days, the gender-reveal party has become the latest trend. Some couples are creating such elaborate celebrations that bakeries are now creating specialty cakes that reveal through confetti or other decorations the sex of the baby.[42] Prior to modern technology, the sex of the baby revealed itself at the birth. With the introduction of testing technology, such as amniocentesis, and then with the ubiquitous use of ultrasounds, it has become common for couples to identify the sex of their baby in their second trimester of pregnancy. Now, we see the sex-identification moment moving to a new phase: the spectacle. A moment, like much of pregnancy, that used to be private for the mother, then private for the couple, is now meant to be a public event for families and friends, with people marketing products, such as invitations or favors, to capitalize on a new consumer moment associated with pregnancy.

Marketers are finding additional ways to encourage couples to mark this passage in their life through consumption. Recognizing the life change that couples are about to face, some hotel chains have introduced special babymoon travel packages. The Starwood Hotel chain offers the "Bundle of Joy Babymoon Package," which includes a tote bag with a teddy bear, "pampering lotions," and a "24-hour Cravings Chef." Sparkling cider and ice cream sundaes have replaced the bedside champagne.[43] Not to be undone, Marriott Hotels offers a Babymoon package that includes a "Musical Energy Balance treatment" and "The Yummy Mummy's Survival Guide book."[44] Couples now only need to go to the website www.babymoonfinder.com to choose between countless luxury packages. Do you want to watch schools of dolphins swim or enjoy a Swedish massage while your baby kicks in your belly? The website details babymoons already taken by celebrities like Kate Hudson and Mariah Carey. The website advertises: "Whatever these parents-to-be are looking for, we hope to find the perfect escape so when baby comes parents are rejuvenated, reconnected, and ready to work!" These babymoons capitalize on the fact that pregnancy, unlike motherhood, has a definite end, so they can create a sense of urgency for couples to take advantage of these services before time runs out.

Once a time for couples to contemplate their changing relationship as their due date nears, marketers have taken this moment and turned it into a time for consumerism. Rituals have become packaged and pregnancy is now treated like a promotional campaign. But the purpose of a promotional campaign is to build excitement and anticipation about an event or the launch of a product. When the campaign is over, people move on. The arrival of a baby, however, is not an ending but a beginning. As the natural waiting period of pregnancy has become a formalized stage centered on consumption, it replaces the organic, natural rituals of preparing for parenthood, setting couples up for their next wave of consumption once the baby arrives.

Outsourcing Parenthood

Expectant mothers are presented with a world of choices, but this comes at a price beyond the cost of the products they buy. Options breed confusion. A healthy, green approach to pregnancy may seem sensible, but do pregnant women really need uniquely formulated yogurt or skin cream? Expectant women now have to evaluate whether each new product is really necessary, or merely a marketing ploy.

The plethora of stores and services now available for pregnant women is the result of a congruence of social and economic changes in society. Many women wait longer to become pregnant. Having had time to complete college and even graduate school, they are more educated than in the past. Products that offer educational elements and unique services appeal to these women, already accustomed to using new technology to research information.

Although women today have more disposable income to purchase pregnancy and baby-related products, money is not the only factor in their purchasing decisions. Since many women have professional careers and fulfilled lives before becoming pregnant, they do not see pregnancy as some did 30 years ago, a time to take a break from the rigors of life. They want to accommodate pregnancy into their already-established routines. They want to continue to have exercise classes and a sex life. Pregnancy and motherhood do not become an integral part of their identity, just another attribute that fits into their lifestyle.

And for many women, these services provide a resource that they need. But in the process, pregnant women are converted into a defined target market, not simply clients but consumers. New trends and "rules" for being pregnant have emerged. Pregnant women are expected to buy trendy clothes that show off their bellies, establish rituals that include painting their pregnant bodies, create blogs that track every moment of their pregnancies, and pose for photographers to capture an image of their belly.

Marketers keep providing new opportunities for women to show off and embrace their pregnancies. Of course, this is not biologically necessary. No studies suggest that baring your belly and promoting your pregnancy leads to healthier babies. But it is a consumer necessity. Many women do not enjoy pregnancy. They feel fat, ugly, and anxious, but the consumer market sees these feelings as a problem and offers their products as solutions.

Depending on experts during pregnancy leads parents to continue to rely on these authorities after the baby is born. There will come a time when a parent is faced with a baby who won't go to sleep, a toddler who resists toilet training, or a recalcitrant teenager who is misbehaving. For all these issues, a cadre of experts is available to help parents get through the process.[45] While parents find valuable the advice of these authorities and the use of these services, they paradoxically become disempowered by falling into a pattern of relying on them. The commercialization of the pregnancy preparation industry has externalized and sold back to mothers the instinct that had emerged naturally during pregnancy, when the woman was the sole connection to her developing child. A mother's intuition is now for sale.

Chapter 7

Womb Time

One pregnant woman told me about her travails to avoid prematurely outing her second pregnancy to her coworkers. She was traveling on business soon after discovering she was pregnant. Typically on these trips, she goes out for dinner and drinks with her colleagues. Her abstinence would seem odd to them, and she was afraid they would guess she was pregnant. So she took the waitress aside, explained her predicament, and asked her that when she ordered a drink, to substitute a nonalcoholic version. Her subterfuge worked, and no one suspected. From that point on, she didn't think twice about enlisting the support of wait staff all across the world. In San Francisco, a particularly excited waitress brought her two "Cosmos." The signs of pregnancy, once confined to the home and often known only to women, are now exposed to the public. People can join in the celebration of pregnancy, as evidenced by the fans of the many reality programs that feature pregnant celebrities. At the same time, marketers are also free to further segment and commoditize the experience of pregnancy. This chapter explores the economic, social, and political consequences of pregnancy moving from a private experience to a publicly celebrated one.

Pregnancy as Performance

Reality television has helped to position the pregnancy experience as a commoditized one by glamorizing and showing off pregnancy. The most obvious example of this is *Pregnant in Heels,* which stars pregnant concierge Rosie Pope, who caters to the needs of rich and pregnant New Yorkers.[1] The opening voiceover has Rosie informing us, "I'm a maternity concierge catering to my clients every need no matter how quirky or impossible and while I don't baby them I always remember they're pregnant in heels." Some of her services include arranging for a pregnant nude photo-shoot on a horse, helping an expectant mother find the perfect personal assistant, or executing one pregnant woman's request that a member of royalty be her baby's godparent (a special English tea has to be arranged).

At the beginning of each program, Pope asserts her authority by having the pregnant mother (and sometimes father) take a "Mommy I.Q." test, where she relishes in the answers they get wrong. By making the moms-to-be feel incompetent early, Pope positions herself as the expert. Pope frequently tells the audience, "I'm hired to help these women but I'm really here to help the babies."[2] She asserts that there are right and wrong ways to raise a child, and she is there to make sure expectant parents get the right start. The program also reinforces that there is a right way to be pregnant. Pope frequently aids women who are not displaying the appropriate levels of enthusiasm for their expectant pregnancies. In one episode, Pope finds herself in a heated argument with a pregnant client that Pope insists is not preparing enough for her baby. By the end of the episode, the woman is grateful to Pope for helping her to prepare for her baby.[3]

By marketing herself as a pregnancy and baby expert, Pope also promotes the need for additional specialists in a variety of services. In most episodes, she is hiring consultants for services one might not even think a consultant exists. She hires consultants to run a focus group to help a couple pick the perfect baby name.[4] In another episode, she hires a sex therapist to assist a woman who feels dissatisfied with her sex life in her third trimester.[5] There is an expert available to solve any potential problem, real or imagined. The symptoms or natural challenges one faces during pregnancy are presented by Pope as a problem that money can solve.

One of the most frequent problems that Pope solves on these programs is the lack of agreement within the couple on how to raise their children. In the episode "Taming the Tiger and the Terror," the mom-to-be wants to raise her child in the "tiger parent" style, an allusion to a recent memoir by an Asian mother about the challenges of using strict parenting to raise children. Pope ends up stepping in with her experts to let the parents see they need to compromise on their approaches. In other episodes, she mediates over the type of birth a couple should have, what religion their child should be, or even who the godparents should be. Decisions, once historically the domain of mostly the males in the family, then a shared couple decision, are now being outsourced to consultants. The ridiculousness of the program is not lost to all viewers. Blogs referencing the show critique even the premise: "In my never ending quest to bring you the absolute worst, most appalling reality shows on television, I present *Pregnant in Heels* on Bravo. Thanks to reader Matt for turning me on to this argument for why rich people are buffoons and shouldn't be allowed to have matches much less children."[6] Yet, the program is in its second season, fueled by a desire on the part of viewers to watch pregnant women, unlimited by financial resources, indulge in glamorous pregnancies.

Reality television programs that feature pregnant main characters also serve to reinforce the notion of pregnancy as a time to indulge in not just food cravings but in merchandise as well. The reality television program *Tia & Tamera* on the Style Network stars Tia and Tamera Mowry, twins who are most famous for their role on the 1990s television sitcom *Sister, Sister*. In this new reality program, they are grown up and showing off their different life stages.[7] Tamera is getting married and planning a huge wedding. Tia is pregnant and an actress. Much of the drama of the program is drawn from the twins' squabbling over who is being the most (or least) supportive during their respective life challenges. Tia, for example, does not want to be maid of honor because her pregnancy gets in the way of her duties. She does not even want to attend a bachelorette party because she thinks it is inappropriate for a pregnant woman to be in the company of a male stripper. Tamera is angry that Tia is not devoting enough time supporting Tamera's wedding plans. At the same time, the program, by positioning through editing these two life changes side by side, equates these two events as having a similar consumer focus. Tamera spends her time before the wedding making decisions that are aesthetic or consumer oriented. She has to decide what products to add to her registry, whether she should wear her hair up or down, and what items to cut back on in order to cut $30,000 off the total cost of her wedding to stay within budget. The show then frames Tia struggling with her own life-stage decisions. She talks about her birth plan and asks, "Do I do a hospital birth?" After she discusses options with her doctor, Tia says, "I really like how she made me feel at ease about the different options . . . I really like what she had to offer, but I'd still like to explore my other options." She then sets up interviews with a midwife and doula, admitting that she "honestly doesn't know the difference between the two." The program frames Tia as shopping for her birth choices in much the way that Tamera is spending for her wedding.

Yet, while many choices can be made for a wedding, choices regarding pregnancy are less necessary than imagined as new consumer options are offered to women. In one episode, Tia breaks down when she finds out that she needs to go on bed rest for the remaining two weeks of her pregnancy. She laments the fact that pregnancy looks so easy for all these people when it's actually not. In fact, while seeming to counter the glorification of pregnancy, Tia is most upset about the loss of control she is experiencing and that this will prevent her from doing all the activities that she needs to do before the baby arrives, in particular, creating the baby's room.[8] She solves her problem by hiring a consultant to buy for the baby.

The second season of *Tia & Tamara* will focus this time on Tamara's pregnancy, but the program is just one of many reality shows that feature a prominent pregnant star. *Bethenny Getting Married's* first season focused on the former *The Real Housewives of New York City* star's pregnancy and wedding plans. Similar to *Tia & Tamara,* the program positions wedding planning next to pregnancy, infusing them both with a consumer mentality. Kim Zolciak, a former star of *The Real Housewives of Atlanta,* also received her own show to showcase a pregnancy and wedding plans in *Don't Be Tardy for the Wedding. The Rachel Zoe Project* earned its highest ratings during an episode in which Zoe gave birth.[9] Tori and Dean's popularity on their reality show *Tori & Dean: Home Sweet Hollywood* on the Oxygen Network centers in part on her pregnancy. She is currently in the sixth season of the program and expecting her fourth child. Working to become pregnant can itself be an entire show as evidenced by the popularity of *Giuliana and Bill* on the Style network, currently completing its fifth season, which focuses mainly on her struggles with infertility. Viewers have watched the couple try to get pregnant, go through in vitro fertilization, suffer a miscarriage, and then hire a surrogate. The couple has just announced an arrangement with a surrogate.

The pregnancy storyline has been proven to work with fans. MTV executives are excited about the ability to capitalize on the pregnancy of one of their lead stars, Nicole Polizzi "Snookie," from the *Jersey Shore.* She is set to star in her own spin-off series, *Snooki and JWoww.* Although *Jersey Shore* is still quite popular, its ratings have dipped, and this pregnancy has been seen as a way to refresh the brand.[10] Kendra Wilkinson, formerly on *The Girls Next Door,* which chronicled Hugh Hefner's life and girls, received her own spin-off when she became engaged and announced she was pregnant.

Once these celebrity reality stars become pregnant, the core biological experience is put aside in favor of the commoditized experience, with a focus on shopping for themselves and their babies. This may be partly due to the medium of television, which biases visually exciting images that not only entertain audiences but also keep them in the mood to shop.[11] It simply is not interesting to watch a pregnant woman have quiet moments of internal connection to her fetus, but it is entertaining to watch her buy for one.

These reality programs and stars further promote the commercialization of pregnancy and birth by granting celebrity interviews that celebrate their pregnancies and then investing in consumer lines to offer endless products for women both during pregnancy and after. Tia Mowry has released an advice book called *Oh, Baby!* The book includes a "Hot Mama" chapter offering advice as to what to wear to remain sexy while pregnant. Kendra Wilkinson created her own book, *Sliding into Home,* and endorsed "Abdominal Cuts," a weight-loss pill. She now has a sequel book out, *Cribs, Cocktails, and Getting my Sexy Back,* which acknowledges her struggles with weight and postpartum depression while still selling sexiness as a solution for women. And pregnancy is only the start of what follows: a business of marketing their babies to sell products. Selling baby photos is big business. The recent photo of Jessica Simpson's infant daughter supposedly brought in $800,000.[12] Victoria Beckham's nine-month old was offered a modeling contract from an online gift store.[13] There are also clothing lines for children. Kourtney Kardashian opened a children's boutique store. Tori Spelling partnered with a company to create the children's clothing line Little Maven.[14] Pregnancy has not simply become a moment that leads to the birth of a child, but the birth of an industry.

"A Little Bit Pregnant": Segmenting Pregnancy

The commoditization of pregnancy as evidenced by celebrity reality stars and the number of products, experts, and services geared toward pregnancy has brought with it a segmentation of the process. At the turn of the 20th century, motherhood became scientifically managed. Experts endorsed the most efficient ways of feeding, toilet training, and breaking bad habits. "Educated mothers in the early 1900s employed quantitative jargon (precise weights and measures; IQs) in referring to their children," writes historian Shari Thurer. "Motherhood, as we have seen, was upgraded to a profession. It was now thought to be lawful, ruled-bound, embodying a body of scientific knowledge that had to be mastered."[15] Today, this maternal Taylorism has crept into the prenatal period. A long popular aphorism, "You can't be a little bit pregnant," is no longer true. New infertility treatments allow women to be just barely pregnant when sperm is implanted (intra-uterine insemination), to a little more pregnant when embryos are implanted (in vitro fertilization), to fully pregnant when hormone tests detect that a woman's body has accepted the embryo. Once this process is segmented, each portion becomes a separate target market, each with its own products and campaigns.

TLC's online show *A Conception Story* follows the journey of women trying to get pregnant.[16] The show is gaining attention not for its subject matter, which is no longer shocking to people, but for its partnership. Its sponsor is First Response, the maker of both ovulation and pregnancy test kits, which are both widely featured on the program. In this relationship, brands are associated with a time of life that used to be considered private. The featured women discuss their sometimes-difficult efforts to get pregnant and how they use the First Response products. One woman lays out on her floor her urine-stained test kit to show how she has been tracking her ovulation cycle. Another woman admits she is still taking the home pregnancy test despite her doctor informing her that her blood test shows a negative result because she trusts First Response more.

This show has moved beyond celebrating pregnancy to fixate on the moment of discovering one is pregnant, and the central role First Response plays in that discovery. Most products advertised on television unjustifiably tout their essential nature in everyday life, and as this book has discussed previously, the invention of these tests have given women a new degree of power and autonomy in family planning. However, now that First Response has become the star of its own program—the women on the show change, but the kits are always there—the product is made to seem like a necessary component of becoming pregnant. Technology replaces a once-natural waiting period with a more precise method that must be purchased. While women having difficulty conceiving may benefit from this technology, these products are marketed to all women, making them the new environmental norm.

For those women who are not ready to embark on pregnancy but who want to ensure their biological capability to do so when they are ready, they can now freeze their eggs. A newer phenomenon emerging is that parents of daughters in their 30s are paying for the egg storage.[17] While at one time in history, parents of daughters focused on producing a sizable dowry to secure a suitable mate, now, the ability to separate reproductive ability from mate selection provides parents with a new opportunity: harnessing the eggs to expand the length of time a daughter will be able to procreate.

Once pregnant, companies are just waiting to offer expectant couples opportunities to engage in the marketplace. In 2011, Facebook added an option to indicate "Expecting" on your Facebook page under "Family."[18] Couples were already attempting to announce their emerging family by creating separate pages for their fetuses. This move, though, becomes not simply a way to let friends and family know your life-changing news, but also serves as a signal for companies that are just as interested in this information.

The segmentation of pregnancy allows companies to target different markets within a group of pregnant women. *American Baby* magazine is now customizing its online magazines depending on the stage you are in during your pregnancy or new motherhood. A woman in her third month of pregnancy will have different articles and features than a woman in her seventh month of pregnancy. The magazine sees this as a response to millennials' desires for customization.[19] Millennials, born on or after 1982, are accustomed to being a target audience. In *Millennials Rising,* Neil Howe and William Strauss discuss how this group has been the target of marketers since birth. It is no wonder that in 2012, during their prime child-bearing years, Millennials would expect companies to cater to their specific needs.[20]

Car companies are quickly recognizing the power of this potential market with an increase in commercials appealing to the pregnant market. The Nissan Zero ad for an electric car highlights the number zero to illustrate how using less can do more. Featured prominently in the commercial is a pregnant woman's belly as a symbol for purity and for potential. This commercial links the car and pregnancy to anticonsumption, ironic considering how much time and energy companies spend on targeting the pregnant woman. In a commercial for Volkswagen's Routan minivan, Brooke Shields's voiceover implies that this family car is so wonderful that it is making people rush to get pregnant in order to be able to attain the car. "And with advances in fertility drugs, cyber adoption, even reverses in vasectomies, more and more people are having babies simply for the love of German engineering." The humor, of course, derives from the fact that one would never have a child just to get a car, while reassuring expectant couples that they can still have a great car when becoming parents. A Nissan Maxima car commercial shows a man just finding out that he is going to become a father. He walks outside and watches his car transform from a two door to a four door but still looking sporty. The voiceover says "Innovation for Daddy. Innovation for all." A Chevy Cruze commercial also features a pregnancy as a main component of the commercial. There is an expectant couple looking and rejecting potential houses. They use the car to travel between houses and eventually realize that the first house they saw is the one that they want. Theoretically, the car makes them see that the grass is not always greener on the other side. They learn that though they may need to sacrifice some desires, they can still be happy. All these commercials link sacrifice and pregnancy. In fact, researchers consistently conduct studies that indicate that parents are less happy than other people.[21] Adjusting to the sacrifice that comes with parenting has long been a natural process that begins during pregnancy. Now companies offer their products as the solution. Instead of looking internally for contentment, the purchase of a new car can offer fulfillment, according to these ads.

At the same time, some companies are moving beyond simply selling products for pregnant woman, but using the pregnancy experience to position consumption in new ways. In an article published in the *New York Times Magazine,* reporter Charles Duhigg uncovered a strange relationship between the Target department store and pregnant women. Target hired data experts to cull information from Target shoppers to create a pregnancy-prediction model. Since Target recognized that pregnancy was a moment where people increased and changed their spending habits, suddenly needing a new array of products, the earlier they could lure them to the store with coupon rewards, the better they can lock them in as a consumer for life. Target found that with this new data, they could identify pregnant women even before they had outed themselves to friends and family as pregnant. Target had to create a strategy where they slowly introduced coupons related to pregnancy so as to not spook pregnant women who didn't want Target to acknowledge their pregnancies before they had.[22] The consumption patterns of pregnancy have become so pervasive that corporations can identify pregnant women before they have made their pregnancies public. Yet, they have to cover up this knowledge because to reveal it would also reveal the unsettling truth that the pregnancy experience has become an experience of consumption. It is creepy to these women because we still think of pregnancy as being internal and that the giving of life should be beyond consumption and instead, Target had revealed it is just another opportunity for marketing.

Pregnant and Marketable

Once pregnant women become a target audience, television networks have to work harder to find niches within this group. Depiction of pregnancy has become so popular and normalized that for networks to gain attention and audience, they are taking pregnancy to the extreme. A new array of shows focuses on unusual pregnancies. *Make Room for Multiples* (TLC) features women giving birth to twins, triplets, quadruplets, and more, *Babies: Special Delivery* (Discovery Health) focuses on traumatic deliveries, *Deliver Me* (Discovery Health) follows the events within an ob-gyn practice, and *House of Babies* (Discovery Health) portrays the midwife experience. The popular programs *I'm Pregnant and . . .*, *I didn't Know I was Pregnant,* and *Sixteen and Pregnant* all follow women who do not have a traditional, normalized pregnancy. These shows are successful precisely because of their contrary portrayals of the ideal pregnancy.

I'm Pregnant and . . . focuses on dysfunctional or nonnormalized pregnant women: hoarders, alcoholics, strippers, obese, imprisoned, or homeless women.[23] Occasionally, the featured women have simply made an unusual life choice, such as the episode "I'm Pregnant . . . and a Nudist." She describes her baby shower as typical "other than the fact that some of us were half naked or fully naked." This is atypical for the program. In most episodes, the pregnant woman is suffering physically, emotionally, or psychologically. Sometimes, the woman is burdened by an illness that prevents her from fully enjoying her pregnancy. "Pregnant with an Obsessive Compulsive Disorder (OCD)" follows a pregnant woman who is afraid of germs. Her condition makes her baby shower, in contrast to the nudist, a frightening place where she only eats from the center of her cake and remains physically isolated from her guests. She refuses her OCD medication to protect her baby but suffers through her pregnancy because of it. In other cases, the women have careers that do not seem compatible with pregnancy, such as "I'm Pregnant and a Trucker" or "I'm Pregnant and a Stripper." The stripper explains that she had to give up her job once she started showing. Her family is struggling financially, and she feels pressure to lose all her pregnancy weight quickly so she can begin working again. At other times, women suffer from addictions such as crystal meth or alcohol. Although the imprisoned woman takes responsibility for her actions and is shown caring about her baby, viewers see her wearing handcuffs while she travels to the doctor's office. Each episode reassures audiences that these women are still good moms or have the potential to be great moms if circumstances were different. The program lumps together dysfunction, addiction, disability, and difference as forces that prevent them from fully enjoying their pregnancies.

I Didn't Know I was Pregnant uses recreations and interviews to dramatize stories of women who manage to go 10 months unaware they are carrying a child.[24] These women explain why they thought it unlikely they were pregnant. Many had been taking birth control pills and had regular menstrual cycles. Women and their husbands testify that their bellies never grew significantly and that they never gained much weight. Viewers are left to wonder whether the women have some psychological block that prevented them from recognizing their own pregnancy. The program contrasts the complete surprise these women experience when they go into labor with the culture's fascination of every stage of pregnancy. The show pities these women because they were robbed of the experience of taking part in the rituals of pregnancies. For this program, giving birth without having reveled in the pregnancy seems to be a miracle itself.

Not long ago, teenaged pregnancy was a hushed topic, and unmarried pregnant teens were hidden from public view. Today, MTV's *Sixteen and Pregnant* uses pregnant teenagers as its stars, as each episode follows a teen's last few months of pregnancy and initial weeks with her newborn.[25] The program has reached such popularity that it inspired MTV to create the spin-off show *Teen Moms,* which follows the lives of some of the *Sixteen and Pregnant* stars after the birth of their babies. Although some critics have reproached the program for glorifying pregnant teenagers, the network takes credit for the show contributing to a decline of teen pregnancy.[26] According to MTV, watching the misery these teens face with a newborn may be a great form of birth control.

A closer viewing of the program, however, reveals that the duration of their pregnancies is perhaps the happiest time for these girls. While pregnant, they engage in the same rituals that have become the norm for pregnant women. Although it is clear that many of the girls are in a precarious financial situation, have tentative relationships with the fathers of their babies, and have strained or outright dysfunctional relationships with their own family, they embrace the pregnant experience as a positive force in their lives. The girls show off their ultrasounds, have baby showers, buy clothes and other products for their expectant baby, and engage in other rituals like baby belly art and pregnancy photography. In one episode, a girl's parents refuse to throw her a baby shower, arguing that her situation is not one to celebrate, but her boyfriend's parents step in to give her a shower instead.[27] Her situation is atypical, though, as most episodes show girls' parents (often single mothers themselves) throwing baby showers and helping their daughters embrace the pregnant experience, though it is clear that they wish they were celebrating under different circumstances. Despite some uncomfortable pregnancy symptoms and many complaints about weight gain, the girls look good pregnant. They often remain in their regular clothes, only resorting to a maternity wardrobe when they are close to their due date. The opening sequence includes an animated sketch of a girl wearing fashionable teen clothing but displaying a characteristic belly bump. From the moment a girl gives birth, however, the program takes a downward turn, as she struggles to cope with a newborn. The contrast between the travails of teen motherhood and the celebratory experience of pregnancy encourages a disconnect between the two inherently coupled events.

These programs illustrate the segmentation of the pregnancy market that networks have created to differentiate their shows. Programs that highlight unusual pregnancies reinforce for pregnant viewers at home the notion that they should be thankful they can experience their pregnancies in a complete and satisfying way. While they may experience some uncomfortable side effects, at least they are not in prison, preparing to birth multiples, are too young to raise a baby, or have missed the experience altogether.

Outing Pregnancy

The commoditization of pregnancy has set up contradictions in the realms of work and law and has complicated the power women have over their bodies. The consumer expectation of entitlement to a pregnancy lifestyle carries over to an anticipation of special treatment within work and legal environments. Simultaneously, the shift of pregnancy to the public sphere creates a desire for full participation without restrictions. This paradox creates opposing needs and desires for pregnant women, forcing the law to catch up with social reality.

In the 1905 *Muller v. Oregon* case, the courts penalized a man for overworking his pregnant employee. In her book *Origins,* Annie Murphy Paul rightly contrasts the *Muller* decision with today's attitude that pregnancy does not need to slow women down. Paul finds this increased expectation for women to do more while pregnant to be its own burden.[28] In 1978, the newly created Pregnancy Discrimination Act required employers to treat pregnant workers the same as others. Now, a growing number of women are filing suits for pregnancy discrimination. The Equal Employment Opportunity Commission (EEOC) reports that discrimination claims have risen 39 per cent over the last 10 years.[29] In 2010, there were over 6,000 suits filed under federal law.[30] Accommodations of pregnant workers jobs once defined as masculine, such as police officer, firefighter, and construction, and barred to women, are now expected to be available to women throughout their pregnancies. After a vocal backlash, a U.S. military commander was forced to rescind an order that punished women who became pregnant while on active duty.[31] In 2002, Verizon paid about $49 million to settle a class action suit with the EEOC, the largest payment in history related to pregnancy discrimination.[32]

In other cases, courts have ruled against the protected status of pregnant women. In 2009, the Supreme Court concluded that AT&T did not have to retroactively provide former employees with higher pensions because they were denied employment and pay prior to the 1978 Act.[33] In a closely watched case against Bloomberg, L.P., in which Bloomberg founder and

New York City Mayor Michael Bloomberg was forced to testify, women attempted to file a class action suit in 2007, arguing that the company discriminates against pregnant women by excluding them from important meetings, reducing their pay, and denying them advancement once pregnant. The courts ultimately ruled against the claim in 2011 by claiming that companies have no legal obligation to provide people with a "work-life balance." The women, they argued, were punished no more than anyone else taking a lengthy leave.[34] In May 2012, members of the House of Representatives in Congress proposed the Pregnant Workers Fairness Act, meant to strengthen protections for pregnant women in the workplace.[35] Today, as pregnant women enjoy a public lifestyle where their pregnancies are treated as special and a variety of services have sprouted up to meet their needs, they are demanding a work environment that also matches their expectations. Commercial environments have already begun to accommodate pregnant women (some chain stores even provide their own parking spots) but work environments, filled with political and economic challenges, are lagging.

Fox News commentator Megyn Kelly received attention on the blogosphere and earned a spot on *The Daily Show* when, after taking three months off for maternity leave, she lashed out at radio talk show host Mike Gallagher. Gallagher had wondered on his program how long Ms. Kelly would be gone from her job and criticized maternity leave as "a racket."[36] Critics accused Kelly of hypocrisy, as she had previously derided maternity leave and pregnancy discrimination as liberal policies, while others praised her new support for working mothers. Rather than retreat from the public during pregnancy, women are now actively advocating within the public sphere for both accommodations and the right to remain within the workforce. The power that women have, however, is being compromised by others expecting to share a part of the public pregnancy.

Fetal Power

During the Renaissance, theories of maternal impressions, including reading and eating habits, emerged. Women were encouraged to adapt their pregnant behavior in order to influence their fetus.[37] However, their primary concern must have been their own survival during childbirth, as maternal death was common. Ironically, though women in the Western world enjoy much higher survival rates today, many remain anxious about whether their behavior will harm their fetus throughout their pregnancy.

As new technologies make the fetus more visible, the public has become consumed with protecting this fetus from any imagined harm. The 17th-century warnings to women to avoid bad dreams for fear of creating an ugly baby may seem laughable today, but our own long lists of "dos and don'ts" for pregnant women may seem just as silly in the future. New concerns arise with each passing day. A recent study warns that pregnant women need to curtail their intake of sugar for fear of causing their fetus to crave sweets and condemning it to a lifetime of obesity.[38]

Certainly, scientific research should alert the public to actual dangers to the fetus. Unfortunately, even multiple studies, let alone a single one, do not often provide definitive results. Despite this, commercial news that traffics in a culture of fear as well as new social media often disseminate this information instantaneously, so pregnant women read about "Female Troubles for Wildlife Raise Human Worries"[39] on the Internet one day and hear about the dangers of fish on cable news the next. The womb, once thought to be the ideal protector of the fetus, now suddenly seems precarious. In one restaurant in Manhattan, waiters had to memorize which of the 180 cheeses they serve are safe for pregnant women to eat.[40] Perhaps these warnings do save the occasional fetus from harm, but at what cost to the mother? Now that pregnancy warnings are well publicized and have become common knowledge, pregnant women frequently complain about the judgment they receive from friends and strangers.

Despite technological advances in maternal care, the culture of pregnancy has reverted to a state where any action a pregnant woman performs may have irrevocable and dangerous outcomes for the fetus. While some women spend their pregnancies immersed in anxiety, others go to the opposite extreme. They refuse to adapt their lifestyle to their pregnancy: some engage in extreme sports, while others keep their physically strenuous jobs as ballet dancers or even opera singers.[41] An Iraq War correspondent celebrated her pregnancy with a baby shower in Baghdad. Although she took leave for the baby's birth, she chose not to change her behavior while pregnant. Others, however, did force changes on her; for instance, the U.S. military did not want to take her up on a Black Hawk helicopter.[42] Although an abundance of pregnancy information and advice is available, a lack of context prevents sifting out the useful from the impractical.

The expansion of the sphere of control does not stop at the father. Through popular culture, the public increasingly is commenting on and controlling the language of pregnancy, leading to control over the pregnancy itself. As friends and family share sonograms in their blogs, Facebook status, tweets, and multimedia texts, the fetus becomes an iconic image. Popular culture has begun to co-opt the meaning of the word "fetus." Less than 10 years ago, only medical professionals and women referring to the physical development of their pregnancy used the term, but now it has become part of the everyday language of television programs to refer to immaturity. In an episode of *Grey's Anatomy*, Alex calls George a "fetus" for dwelling over complications he encounters with his friend Meredith after sleeping with her.[43] In the comedy *30 Rock*, Jenna receives collagen injections and asks her colleague Liz if she looks more youthful. Liz's responds, "No, younger even, you look like a fetus."[44]

William Safire, in his *New York Times Magazine* column "On Language," noted the emergence of the phrase "belly bump" to describe the pregnant belly.[45] "A new sense of an old word has been born and appears to be here to stay," he wrote. "Needless embarrassment has been replaced by pride in pregnancy, and the unmistakable sign of impending childbirth is called a bump." In 2008, the *Urban Dictionary* declared the "baby bump" the word of the day.[46] The physical components of pregnancy are entering our everyday language.

These days the image of the fetus is used to advertise products not related to pregnancy.[47] A commercial for Volvo shows an ultrasound video of a fetus waving while the announcer asks, "Is something inside telling you to buy a Volvo?" A controversial ad for fast food chain Carl's Jr. has a fetus in the womb threatening his mom that he'll "come out early" if she keeps eating spicy food.[48] Apparently, babies are no longer cute enough to sell goods; as the signifier of the baby image has been exhausted, the public use of the fetus replaces it. With this comes a redefining of the word. Once meant to distinguish a pre-baby in the womb that needs its mother's physical body to survive, "fetus" now refers to an extreme version of a baby. The new meaning brings with it changes in the politics of defining power over pregnancy.

In Phoenix, Candace Wilkinson stirred controversy when she entered a high-occupancy commuter lane that required two people in a vehicle.[49] She claimed that, because she was pregnant, her fetus counted as another person. Public outcry and the law quickly rejected her argument, but her attempt seems less far-fetched in light of the increased visibility of the fetus.

The public consumption of fetal images has led to competing groups of varying political persuasions using those images to advocate for their causes. The line of defining personhood shifts when the public can see the fetus as an image separate from its environment. Pro-life organizations have begun to capitalize on the concept that the fetus deserves its own human rights. Church groups use ultrasound to encourage women to bond with their fetus and dissuade them from considering abortion.[50] Randall Terry, an ardent antiabortion activist and sometimes political candidate, made waves over his plans to use fetus ads in antiabortion commercials during the 2012 Super Bowl.[51]

In a society infatuated with the pregnancy culture and enamored with the fetus icon, abortion foes have found that these developments can help their cause.[52] Some states are following through with this approach. Oklahoma created a law, later blocked by courts, that had forced women wanting an abortion to first obtain an ultrasound and have described to them the development of their fetus.[53] Virginia ran into controversy over a bill that required doctors to perform vaginal ultrasounds to women considering abortion. In Alabama, a bill mandated that the fetus be seen in the "clearest image," which implied that women must receive a vaginal ultrasound and be forced to face the screen for viewing it. Idaho, Texas, Pennsylvania, and Mississippi are just some of the other states considering laws like these.[54]

Fetal rights is a slippery slope, leading states to prosecute pregnant women for health practices deemed dangerous to their fetus, including drug use, alcohol abuse, and smoking.[55] A *New York Times* article details how laws that originated to protect pregnant women against criminals, are now being used to prosecute pregnant women themselves for endangering their fetuses through drug use.[56] Campaigns to persuade women not to smoke use pictures of a fetus to guilt mothers into behaving. One study suggests: "The types of antismoking messages that I have analyzed, which portray fetuses as independent agents and women who smoke as bad mothers, pose more harm to pregnant women than good to their babies-to-be. Mixing health advice with moral judgments against smoking supports the perception that public intervention into the maternal-fetal relationship on behalf of the fetus is socially, medically, and legally justified."[57]

Scientists are attempting to determine what a fetus feels within the womb. In some studies, a doctor measures fetal pain by evaluating how the fetus avoids or responds to scalpels. These studies are now possible because of the development of visualization technologies. States increasingly are considering legislation that takes fetal pain into account. Nebraska has already passed a law restricting abortions after 20 weeks because of fetal pain.[58] Senator Sam Brownback (Kansas) has introduced a bill titled the Unborn Child Pain Awareness Act, which would require that a fetus be offered anesthesia before any medical procedures. Some researchers are suggesting that fetuses should be given pain relief before a difficult birth.[59]

While mothers often have sought to make their children's lives more comfortable, this impulse is now extending into the prenatal period. The desire for comfort is being projected into the womb. Pro-choice groups struggle within this new semantic environment. Focused on the rights of a woman to make decisions about her body, the movement faces a popular culture that celebrates the fetus as an autonomous being and an expanding market that involves others during pregnancy.

Pregnancy Backlash

As others, including the fetus, gain attention and power over pregnancy, pregnant women themselves begin to lose both political standing and social status. Resentment has begun to surface against pregnant women. A popular YouTube video titled "Pregnant Women are Smug" mocks the special status that pregnant women claim for themselves. The comedy songwriting duo who go by the name Garfunkel and Oates strum a guitar and sing lyrics like, "This whole world that you are enjoying/Makes you really annoying." With over two million views, the song critiques pregnant women for the clichés and self-importance they adopt when expecting.

A story on *Cosmopolitan*'s website titled "Pregnant Chicks Who Brag too Much" compiles a list of rants from readers about the behavior of their pregnant friends. One woman described an incident of overreaction. She was heating up a can of spaghetti for herself. Her pregnant friend, standing nearby, left the room because "she didn't want her baby to be anywhere near foods with preservatives." Another complained about a pregnant woman who felt entitled to cut in front of her in line at the gym.[60] Tirades in the blogosphere complain about spots in parking lots designated as "stork parking." As New York City considers a bill that would allow women with difficult pregnancies to be allowed special parking privileges, blogs have responded with headlines like, "Should You Get Special Privileges for Getting Knocked Up?"[61]

It may be surprising to some that backlash to pregnancy is nothing new. In the Medieval period, to be pregnant was to remind others that a woman had engaged in a sexual act, a disturbing image to those devoted to Christianity.[62] In the Early Modern era, unmarried mothers often abandoned their babies or risked being ostracized.[63] Poor pregnant women were resented in the 1930s for the additional burden they represented within a society in the midst of the Great Depression.[64] More recently, Vice President Dan Quayle infamously criticized fictional character Murphy

Brown in 1992 for having a child out of wedlock. All of these examples illustrate reactions to a perceived threat to the social order. It is unclear what threat today's pregnant woman poses to society. Perhaps some are reacting to the commoditization of the pregnant experience, or the identity politics that treats pregnancy as a protected status, or simply the movement of pregnancy from the private to the public sphere. Whatever the reason, it is the woman carrying a pregnancy who becomes the target.

Conclusions

In her now classic book *Birth as an American Rite of Passage*, Robbie E. Davis-Floyd writes of the technocratic birth, criticizing how the birth process: ". . . has been culturally transformed in the United States into a male-dominated initiatory rite of passage through which birthing women are taught about the superiority, the necessity, and the 'essential' nature of the relationship between science, technology, patriarchy, and institutions."[65] Davis-Floyd laments how the medical profession wrested control of the birth process from women, yet the commoditization of pregnancy culture seems to encourage women to willingly give up control. When pregnancy becomes performance for a public audience, women cede control not only of the physical process but also its symbolic environment, which distracts them from determining what their pregnancy means. Their choices of pregnancy products become trivial, and their identities become wrapped up in branded categories.

While women dwell over whether they are more of a "yummy mummy" or "earth mom," they have less time to consider the deeper questions of loss of self and sacrifice that come with motherhood. Conceivably, ovulation tests can help retrieve pregnancy from the domain of medical professionals and freezing eggs can allow women their own reproductive timetable. Both could reinforce the woman as the primary arbiter of her own body. This would recall earlier periods when a woman's instincts governed the process and a network of women assisted her in her pregnancy and birth. Instead, corporations have retained the power for themselves.

Women have the illusion of controlling their pregnancies, but only through making choices of which product to buy or activity to indulge in, often with the profits going back to companies that continue to make even more pregnancy products and services to sell. Most of these products are not harmful in and of themselves and the corporations producing them do so not with malice. Yet, these products help to create a branded lifestyle, and pregnancy itself runs the risk of resembling just another fad.

The focus on branding pregnancy also has economic and political consequences. While, on the consumption side, there is this desire by companies to create a consumer market and environment for pregnant women, on the production side, there is a resistance by companies to accommodate the pregnancy lifestyle. The increased use of the image of the fetus in public also has led some to reposition these same images as a threat to a women's right of control over the fetus in her womb. The increased commoditization of pregnancy opens a new door into the process. It allows women to invite others into the experience and permits glimpses into the pregnancies of strangers. However, once this door is open, marketers and other groups will invite themselves in as well, resulting in clashes as different voices mingle within the womb.

Chapter 8

The Big Let-Down

Changes in media environments are reshaping how society understands pregnancy. Media technology continuously impacts how people see their environments. However, people are slow to notice these gradual changes, their consequences, or even society's ability to influence them. Ultrasound technology allows doctors and parents-to-be to peer into the fetus with surprising clarity and to retain the images. The Internet, cell phones, and cameras encourage people to document pregnancy closer and more frequently than ever before. Social media technologies permit expectant couples to share their pregnancies, advice, and joy with distant family and strangers that they may never meet. The public has become a pregnant voyeur during what was once a private time for a woman and her fetus. Women are now free to be pregnant in public, even wearing a bikini if they choose. On a deeper level, they can be open about their pregnancies, feelings, and demands. The commoditization of the pregnant experience, however, is the price we pay for this new freedom.

From the time that a woman conceives, marketers have ensured that her next nine months will be a consumer's paradise. Though most doctors make women wait until they are about eight weeks along before they begin their pregnant medical journey, the consumer market is happy to immediately allow women to "feel" pregnant. They have advice books to buy, websites to sign onto for their daily fetus reports, and pregnancy-friendly natural cosmetics to purchase. They can begin shopping for fashion-forward maternity clothing, sign up for prenatal yoga, get pregnancy massages, and consider cord blood banking. In the last trimester, baby product registries, belly molding, pregnancy photos, classes on CPR, childbirth, breast-feeding, and child care are all available. So many choices are available to women that baby planners often are booked to help them negotiate the process. Throughout her pregnancy, a woman can listen to her baby's heartbeat with her personal stethoscope and keep a fetal journal and picture album. She can write a blog promoting her pregnancy, where she can solicit potential names from friends and strangers alike. Finally, she can spend a portion of her day stimulating the fetus in her womb with music and other products marketed to improve fetal development. One website titled "I'm Bored in Here! Games for Baby in the Womb" projects a mother's restlessness of waiting onto the fetus.[1]

The segmentation of the pregnant experience allows marketing to expand beyond pregnant women themselves. Expectant dads now have a range of activities offered just for them. They have their own advice books, create their own blogs, have their own expectant dad classes, and even command honored roles in baby showers. They are encouraged to let the fetus hear their voice, be a regular presence during ultrasounds, and to think of ways to support their pregnant partners. Husbands buy push presents to give to their wives during birth, apparently because the child alone is no longer enough of a gift. Even those not physically present can participate. With surrogate pregnancies, couples, both straight and gay, can vicariously experience the pregnancy and birth of their children. Pregnancy has transformed from a physical state to a lifestyle, which expands its domain beyond the body of the pregnant woman.

A new test allows men to examine their fertility from the privacy of their own home,[2] and scientists are currently testing a birth control pill for a man, which works by reducing the male sperm count. Though the pill shifts the burden of birth control from women to men, it also precludes women from controlling fertility while encumbering them with the responsibility of carrying a resulting pregnancy.[3] A burgeoning fathers' rights movement, primarily concerned with child custody cases, has turned its attention to pregnancy, advocating for men to have a role in the decision of whether to terminate a pregnancy.[4]

Today, expectant fathers regularly attend their partner's first ultrasound. Just as new technologies offer the same access to fathers as mothers in seeing their fetus, new social conceptions of pregnancy allow them greater access to pregnancy culture. If fathers can be more involved in viewing their developing child, why would they then be satisfied with being passive observers to that development? Books and websites targeting expectant fathers offer advice and exercises they can conduct to bond with the fetus. Women now receive pregnancy advice from not only their mothers, friends, and doctors, but also their male partners, armed with a wealth of information from books, blogs, and websites. Though her womb carries the fetus, a woman is no longer the sole arbiter of her pregnancy.

Pregnancy used to be measured by natural time, a process that could not be rushed and was beyond the control of people or technology. This was a source of frustration to philosophers and doctors in antiquity (sometimes one and the same), as they had difficulty predicting the exact duration of a pregnancy. Today, the pregnant experience is one of the few times in modern life that can't be tampered with, requiring a rushed populace to listen to nature. As technocratic culture constantly seeks new efficiencies, pregnancy can be a refreshing change of pace that cannot be altered, though some have tried. Recently, celebrities have popularized the notion of the elective Cesarean section, allowing women to essentially schedule the birth of their child rather than wait for nature to determine when labor begins.[5] The pop star Victoria Beckham, also known as Posh Spice, was the inspiration for the phrase "too posh to push" after she chose to give birth via C-section. Advocates argue that C-sections are no more dangerous than natural births, though it does involve major surgery. The perceived desire to shorten the duration of pregnancy has become so great that the nonprofit group March of Dimes recently launched HBWW (healthy babies are worth the wait), a public awareness campaign that encourages women to carry their pregnancies to term.[6] Past generations would marvel that our culture would need a campaign to influence women on how long to be pregnant.

When the outside world defines the pace of pregnancy and anyone can buy a piece of the pregnant lifestyle, the mother-fetal relationship changes. Debates already are emerging about the medical consequences of this shift. Women used to dream about their future baby, but now they can pay for a personalized 4-D ultrasound experience to see the emerging features of their child. Unsure of the potential harmful effects of these ultrasounds, the FDA has issued warnings that pregnant women should not seek nonmedical ultrasounds to gather keepsake videos.[7] Beyond medical concerns, the social experiences of pregnancy are also changing. One woman described to me her disappointment in seeing her baby in such detail before the birth. When she finally held her baby, she was shocked at how much the baby looked like its fetal image. For her, the sonogram diminished the birth moment.

Over time, birth has lost much of its mystery. Parents can evaluate the relative health of their baby, its approximate weight, and, earlier than ever before, its sex. Thanks to the widespread use of ultrasound, most parents obtain a representation of their baby before holding the physical being, conforming to the expectations of an image culture. Precision ultrasound becomes yet another distraction. Treated to a captive audience, marketers cannot make babies come faster, but they can make the waiting feel faster. Pregnancy, traditionally a time of internal connection between mother and child, has now become an externalized process that involves others.

Pregnancy used to be a time of preparation and reflection. Before the 20th century, the physical risks of childbirth compelled women to consider the very nature of their own survival. As those risks diminished through the last century, women still wondered how impending motherhood would impact their social and psychological reality. Now that pregnancy is becoming understood as its own phase of life, with commoditized rituals and products, less time is available to ponder the impact of motherhood. Parenthood feels like a sudden shock when compared to the attention showered upon pregnancy. Mayra, a mother and model, remembers her experiences being photographed while pregnant and after the birth of her child. During her pregnancy, Mayra found that she was catered to while on photo shoots in a way that she had never experienced during her previous years as a model. "All of a sudden," she said, "everyone really cares how you feel." Though she had never posed nude before, she felt completely comfortable doing so while pregnant. "I just felt like I was wearing this costume that was my body." The photographs of her posing in ways she would never agree to do before her pregnancy gave her a different perception of herself. "When you are pregnant, you really feel like your body is not your own." A few weeks after she gave birth, she returned for another shoot, posing with her new baby. The difference was startling to her. "I was nude, and this time it was my body again, and it was all distorted. It almost felt damaged to a point, sagging and leaking everywhere, and I had a tear from the birth. I was really uncomfortable." Managing an uncooperative baby and an impatient photographer, Mayra struggled to set up the perfect pose of mother and child. Feeling like a failure, she realized that mother-newborn child images were a fiction. "We often see the beautiful images," she said. "We often see the postpartum images of the beautiful mom and baby, but giving everyone that image of the peaceful mom and baby was really hard to achieve."

Mayra's story illustrates a problem with the extreme celebration and idealization of pregnancy. As pregnancy is relished, less attention is paid to resources devoted to the mother post-birth. In her book *The Immigrant Advantage: What we Can Learn from Newcomers to America about Health, Happiness and Hope*, Claudia Kolker describes the "cuarentena" of Hispanic culture, when women fill the 40 days post-birth with rituals that focus attention on the health and care of the new mother and baby.[8] In the United States, women have nothing akin to these rituals for healthy moms post-birth, let alone mothers who need extra help.

Recently, a few celebrity moms have broken through the façade of perfect parenting to reveal their own struggles with postpartum depression. Brooke Shields wrote in her memoir, *Down Came the Rain*, how she smiled with her newborn daughter while feeling anything but happy.[9] Actress Gwyneth Paltrow also revealed that depression sapped the joy that she was expected to feel after the birth of her second. Revelations such as these from celebrities are an honest and refreshing departure from the usual motherhood-is-no-problem stories.[10] Yet, the length of time it took for both women to self-diagnose their condition reveals an important contradiction. Pregnancy is celebrated as a happy, wonderful experience for women, but the problems that can come during and after birth are pushed to the margins, if they are recognized at all.[11]

Surely, few people have a problem with a society that celebrates the arrival of its newest members. Pregnant women often talk about the kindness and interest that strangers take in their pregnancies. We certainly would not want a return to a time when women were kept hidden, fearing childbirth, with little sense of control over the process. However, with this societal celebration and focus on pregnancy, there is a pressure on women to be happy from the moment of conception. The journey to motherhood requires reflection and sometimes even moments of solemnity, because it involves the loss of a previous life. The physical burden of carrying the pregnancy still remains primarily the role of the mother-to-be. Women still retain the biological responsibility of pregnancy and are left with managing the psychological and physical impact of their bodies postpartum. Women often still face the primary responsibility of caring for the child but are offered few resources to manage that job. The introduction of pregnancy into public culture is not accompanied by an equal sharing and managing of the process. A focus on purchasing and glorifying this stage of life crowds out moments that do not involve consumer action. The consumer pregnancy offers women a way to acknowledge, enjoy, and be public with their pregnancies, but it does not bring real power for a woman to consider what her pregnancy, and her baby, will mean to her life.

Conclusion

The title of this book, *A Womb with a View*, reflects a society busy both peering into pregnancy and projecting onto the fetus, attaching greater significance to this phase of life. As pregnancy moves from a private experience to a public one, others not traditionally involved in pregnancy have become a part of the process. As the fetus gains rights distinct from its mother, governments at the federal, state, and local levels are regulating the treatment of the fetus, and ultimately the pregnancy process itself. Simultaneously, corporations have defined a new segmented target market. None of this is inherently bad. New regulation can provide clarity at times when reproductive technologies create confusion over rights and responsibilities. Companies can supply products and services that many expectant mothers find useful. However, technology brings with it a Faustian Bargain as my mentor, media scholar Neil Postman, used to say. For all the power a new technology provides, it also takes some away.[12] This book did not set out to judge these products or the shift of pregnancy from private to public. Instead, its goal is to bring awareness to how technology and popular culture have influenced how we see pregnancy. Understanding these changes empowers us to think, make informed choices, and retrieve some level of control over this basic human experience.

Notes

Chapter 1 Outing Pregnancy: From Stork to Sonogram

1. Taken from the following websites:

   American Pregnancy Association, http://www.americanpregnancy.org/.
   BabyCenter, L.L.C., http://www.babycenter.com/.
   BYG Publishing, Inc., http://www.bygpub.com/natural/pregnancy.htm.
   Hearst Corporation, http://www.womansday.com/.
   Meredith Corporation, http://www.parents.com/.
   WebMD, L.L.C., http://www.webmd.com/.
   Yahoo Inc., http://www.yahoo.com/.

2. Susan Kuchinskas, "All the World's a GoldenPalace.com," *Internetnews.com*, June 1, 2005, http://www.internetnews.com/ec-news/article.php/3508966/All+the +Worlds+a+GoldenPalacecom.htm.

3. Marshall McLuhan, *Understanding Media: The Extensions of Man* (New York: The New American Library, Inc., 1964).

4. For everyone that agreed to be interviewed for this book, I made an offer to use a pseudonym to preserve their anonymity. Though some preferred to have their real names used, I changed the names of those who did not.

Chapter 2 A Window into the Womb

1. Ned Potter, "Parents Make Facebook Page for Unborn Child: Becomes Online Journal," *ABC News*, June 2, 2011, http://abcnews.go.com/Technology/ facebook-page-unborn-baby-marriah-greene-texas-page/story?id=13734579#. T-BZRvXNmPM.

2. Tina Cassidy, *Birth: The Surprising History of How We are Born* (New York: Atlantic Monthly Press, 2006), 32.

3. Cassidy, *Birth: The Surprising History,* 32–33.

4. Jacques Gélis, *History of Childbirth: Fertility, Pregnancy, and Birth in Early Modern Europe,* Translated by Rosemary Morris (Cambridge, UK: Polity Press, 1991), 62.

5. Gélis, *History of Childbirth,* 19.

6. Ibid., 46.

7. Annie Murphy Paul, *Origins: How the Nine Months before Birth Shape the Rest of Our Lives* (New York: Free Press, 2010).

8. Cristina Mazzoni, *Maternal Impressions: Pregnancy and Childbirth in Literature and Theory* (Ithaca, NY: Cornell University Press, 2002), 16.

9. Jane Sharp, *The Midwives Book or the Whole Art of Midwifery Discovered: Directing Childbearing Women How to Behave Themselves* (London: Printed for Simon Miller, at the Start at the Well End of St. Pauls, 1671, Reprint, New York and London: Garland Publishing, Inc., 1985), 185.

10. Mazzoni, *Maternal Impressions,* 22.

11. Sally G. McMillen, *Motherhood in the Old South: Pregnancy, Childbirth, and Infant Rearing* (Baton Rouge, LA: Louisiana State University Press, 1990), 37.

12. Clare Hanson discusses this theme in her book Clare Hanson, *A Cultural History of Pregnancy: Pregnancy, Medicine and Culture, 1750–2000* (New York: Palgrave MacMillan Press, 2004), 28.

13. Mazzoni, *Maternal Impressions,* 17.

14. Thomas Bull, *Hints to Mothers, for the Management of Health During the Period of Pregnancy, and in the Lying-In Room; With an Exposure of Popular Errors in connection with Those Subjects,* From the 3rd London edition (New York: Wiley & Putnam, 1842), Micropublished in *History of Women* (New Haven, CT: Research Publications, Inc., 1975), 11.

15. Ziv Eisenberg, "Clear and Pregnant Danger: The Making of Prenatal Psychology in Mid-Twentieth Century America, *Journal of Women's History* 22, no. 3 (2010): 112–35.

16. Nicholas J. Eastman, M.D., *Expectant Motherhood* (Boston: Little, Brown, and Company, 1957), 36.

17. Mazzoni, *Maternal Impressions.*

18. Gélis, *History of Childbirth,* 47.

19. Ann Oakley, *The Captured Womb: A History of the Medical Care of Pregnant Women* (New York: Basil Blackwell, Inc., 1984), 18–19.

20. Sharp, *The Midwives Book,* 103–4.

21. W. E. Fothergill, *Manual of Midwifery: For the Use of Students and Practitioners* (New York: The Macmillan Company, 1896), 44–45.

22. Fothergill, *Manual of Midwifery,* 45.

23. Oakley, *The Captured Womb,* 96–97.

24. Sarah A. Leavitt, "'A Private Little Revolution': The Home Pregnancy Test in American Culture," *Bulletin of the History of Medicine* 80, no. 2 (Summer 2006): 322.

25. Rebecca Lipsitz, "Pregnancy Tests," *Scientific American* 283, no. 5 (November 2000): 110.

26. Sarah A. Leavitt, "A Thin Blue Line: A History of the Pregnancy Test Kit," Website produced by the Stetten Museum, Office of NIH History, in cooperation with the Center for History and New Media at George Mason University and its

Exploring and Collecting History Online (ECHO) project, which is funded by the Alfred P. Sloan Foundation, December 2003, http://history.nih.gov/exhibits/thinblueline/index.html.

27. First Response Website, Church & Dwight Co., Inc., http://www.firstresponse.com/index.asp (accessed August 1, 2007).

28. E.P.T. Website, Insight Pharmaceuticals, LLC, http://www.errorprooftest.com./ (accessed August 1, 2007).

29. Leavitt, "A Private Little Revolution," 326.

30. Ibid., 338.

31. Peeonastick.com, http://www.peeonastick.com (accessed June 22, 2012).

32. TwoWeekWAIT.com, http://www.twoweekwait.com/ (accessed June 22, 2012).

33. Leavitt, "A Private Little Revolution," 328.

34. UNfoundation.org press release, October 21, 1999, as reported in "Mexico City: First Female Mayor Prohibits Pregnancy Tests," *Women's International Network News* 26, no. 1 (Winter 2000): 72.

35. Kamau High, "Pregnancy Test's Clearblue Odyssey," *Adweek,* December 18, 2006.

36. Of course, this isn't completely true. While frank discussion of women's sexuality is permissible on programs like *Sex and the City,* ask anyone who has breastfed a baby in public. There are still many aspects of U.S. culture that are more wary about sex in a number of forms.

37. Website of AdRants, http://www.adrants.com/2004/10/pregnancy-test-suspense-sells-harlequin-b.php (accessed August 1, 2007).

38. José Van Dijck, "The Transparent Body: A Cultural Analysis of Medical Imaging," in *In Vivo: The Cultural Mediations of Biomedical Science,* ed. Phillip Thrutle and Robert Mitchell (Seattle: University of Washington Press, 2005), 5.

39. Jenny Carter and Thérèse Duriez, *With Child: Birth through the Ages* (Edinburgh: Mainstream Publishing, 1986), 48–51.

40. Sylvia D. Hoffert, *Private Matters: American Attitudes toward Childbearing and Infant Nurture in the Urban North, 1800–1860* (Chicago: University of Illinois Press, 1989), 73.

41. Spar, *The Baby Business, How Money, Science, and Politics Drive the Commerce of Conception* (Boston: Harvard Business School Publishing, 2006), 12.

42. Hanson, *A Cultural History of Pregnancy,* 47.

43. Cassidy, *Birth: The Surprising History,* 20.

44. Van Dijck, *In Vivo: The Cultural Mediations,* 102–3.

45. Barbara Duden, *Disembodying Women: Perspectives on Pregnancy and the Unborn,* Translated by Lee Hoinacki (Cambridge: Harvard University Press, 1993), 14.

46. Van Dijck, *In Vivo: The Cultural Mediations,* 103.

47. Rebecca Kukla, *Mass Hysteria: Medicine, Culture, and Mothers' Bodies* (New York: Rowman and Littlefield, 2005).

48. For more information on how the ultrasound was marketed to obstetricians in order to encourage its growth, read Janelle Taylor's "A Fetish Is Born: Sonographers and the Making of the Public Fetus," in *Consuming Motherhood,* eds. Janelle S. Taylor, Linda L. Layne, and Danielle F. Wozniak (New Brunswick, NJ: Rutgers University Press, 2004).

49. Her name has been changed to preserve her anonymity.

50. Janelle S. Taylor, "Image of Contradiction: Obstetrical Ultrasound in American Culture," eds. Sarah Franklin and Helena Ragoné Taylor, *Reproducing Reproduction: Kinship, Power and Technological Innovation* (Philadelphia, PA: University of Pennsylvania Press, 1997), 19–22.

51. In the 1960s, the use of a thermal paper printer allowed for ultrasound images to become portable. See Taylor, "A Fetish is Born," 196.

52. Taylor, "Image of Contradiction," 26.

53. Taylor, "A Fetish Is Born," 195.

54. Neela Banerjee, "Church Groups Turn to Sonogram to Turn Women from Abortions," *New York Times,* February 2, 2005, A1, A15.

55. Advertisement for "Fetal Fotos," Stamford and West Hartford Prenatal Imaging Centers, April 2004 mailing.

56. Van Dijck, *In Vivo: The Cultural Mediations,* 4.

57. E. Ann Kaplan explores the disturbing image of the fetus as a person in films such as *Look Who's Talking Too.* See E. Ann Kaplan. *Motherhood and Representation: The Mother in Popular Culture and Melodrama* (New York: Routledge, 1992), 209.

58. The song has gone on to become the theme song to the television program *House.*

59. Michelle Tauber, "The Private World of Katie Holmes," *People Magazine,* April 24, 2006, 69.

60. Taylor, "Image of Contradiction," 26; Taylor, "A Fetish Is Born," 106–7.

61. Marc Santora, "In Fetal Photos, New Developments," *New York Times,* May 17, 2004.

62. A less expensive but a more common method for parents to observe the fetus is through the purchase of a fetal heartbeat monitor.

63. Abby Lippman, "The Genetic Construction of Prenatal Testing: Choice, Consent, or Conformity for Women?" in *Women and Prenatal Testing: Facing the Challenges of Genetic Technology,* eds. Karen H. Rothenberg and Elizabeth J. Thomson (Columbus: Ohio State University Press, 1994), 10.

64. Claudia Wallis, "The Down Dilemma," *Time Magazine,* November 21, 2005, 65.

65. Andrew Pollack, "DNA Blueprint for Fetus Built Using Tests of Parents," *New York Times,* June 6, 2012, http://www.nytimes.com/2012/06/07/health/tests-of-parents-are-used-to-map-genes-of-a-fetus.html?pagewanted=all.

66. Karen Rothenberg, "The Tentative Pregnancy," in *Women and Prenatal Testing: Facing the Challenges of Genetic Technology,* eds. Karen H. Rothenberg and Elizabeth J. Thomson (Columbus: Ohio State University Press, 1994), 261.

67. Elizabeth Weil, "A Wrongful Birth?" *New York Times Magazine,* March 12, 2006. In fact, one of the first cases of this type was in 1966 involving a disabled child (*Gleitman v. Cosgrove,* 49 NJ 22, 227 A.2d 689(1967). The New Jersey Supreme Court decided in favor of defendants (50).

68. Amy Harmon, "Couples Cull Embryos to Halt Heritage of Cancer," *New York Times,* September 3, 2006.

69. Amy Harmon, "Genetic Testing + Abortion=???" *New York Times,* May 13, 2007.

70. Pam Belluck, "Test Can Tell Fetal Sex at 7 Weeks, Study Says," *New York Times,* August 9, 2011.

71. Sarvenaz Zand, "Parents Sue over Pregnancy Test Said to Tell Baby's Sex," ABC News, February 28, 2006, http://abcnews.go.com/Health/story?id=1668125&page=1#.T-Ea6_XNmPM.

72. The Babyplus Company LLC, http://www.babyplus.com/.

73. Make Way for Baby, http://www.makewayforbaby.com/babies/.

74. Pamela Paul, *Parenting Inc.* (New York: Henry Holt, 2008), 95.

75. Paula Gallant Eckard, *Maternal Body and Voice in Toni Morrison, Bobbie Ann Mason, and Lee Smith* (Columbia, Missouri: University of Missouri Press, 2002), 23.

76. Gélis, *History of Childbirth,* 99.

77. Ibid., 103.

78. Hoffert, *Private Matters,* 194.

79. Ibid., 119–20.

80. Carter and Duriez, *With Child: Birth,* 59.

81. Brigitte Jordan, *Birth in Four Cultures: A Crosscultural Investigation of Childbirth in Yucatan, Holland, Sweden, and the United States* (Prospect Heights, IL: Waveland Press, Inc., 1993), 51.

82. Jordan, *Birth in Four Cultures,* 55.

83. Cassidy, *Birth: The Surprising History,* 55–58.

84. Ibid., 62.

85. Ibid., 64–65.

86. Ibid., 199–200.

87. Michel Odent, *The Farmer and the Obstetrician* (New York: Free Association Books, 2002), 102.

88. Elissa Gootman, "Honey, the Baby is Coming; Quick, Call the Photographer," *New York Times,* June 17, 2012, A1, A4, late edition.

89. Karen Springen, "No Candid Camera," *Newsweek,* February 20, 2006, 16.

90. Ibid.

91. Pretty Pushers, http://www.prettypushers.com/.

92. Jed Lipinski, "For a Gallery at the Edge, Fame is Born Tuesday," *New York Times,* October 30, 2011, MS 1, 7.

93. Paul, *Origins: How the Nine Months.*

Chapter 3 It Takes an E-Village

1. "The Gestation Project," www.enjoyyourdigitallife.com (accessed September 21, 2006).

2. Eastman, *Expectant Motherhood,* 3.

3. Gélis, *History of Childbirth,* 66.

4. Rev. Thomas Searle, *A Companion for the Season of Maternal Solicitude* (New York, Moore and Paynel, Clinton Hall, 1834), 21.

5. Hoffert, *Private Matters,* 48.

6. Ibid., 26–31.

7. Carter and Duriez, *With Child: Birth,* 22.

8. Gélis, *History of Childbirth,* 45.

9. Hoffert, *Private Matters,* 3.

10. Carter and Duriez, *With Child: Birth,* 61.

11. Jordan, *Birth in Four Cultures,* 50.

12. Ibid., 50.

13. Carter and Duriez, *With Child: Birth,* 71.

14. Gélis, *History of Childbirth,* 76.

15. Hoffert, *Private Matters,* 16.

16. Ibid., 193.

17. Maternity Center Association, *Routines for Maternity Nursing and Briefs for Mothers Club Talks* (New York: Maternity Center Association, Revised, 1935), 6.

18. Anonymous posting, *Babble Boards: Pregnancy,* http://www.babble.com/ (accessed July 17, 2007).

19. Mary E. Fissell, *Vernacular Bodies: The Politics of Reproduction in Early Modern England* (New York: Oxford University Press, 2004), 14.

20. Ibid., 30.

21. Ibid., 17.

22. Sharp, *The Midwives Book,* 181.

23. Ibid., 188.

24. Paul Starr, *The Creation of the Media: Political Origins of Modern Communications* (New York: Basic Books, 2004), 137–43.

25. Hoffert, *Private Matters,* 10.

26. Ann Hulbert, *Raising America: Experts, Parents, and a Century of Advice about Children* (New York: Alfred A. Knopf, 2003).

27. Julia Grant, *Raising Baby by the Book: The Education of American Mothers* (New Haven: Yale University Press, 1998), 15.

28. Fothergill, *Manual of Midwifery.*

29. Searle, *A Companion for the Season.*

30. Pye Henry Chavasee, *Advice to a Mother on the Management of Her children: And on the Treatment on the Moment of Some of Their More Pressing Illnesses and Accidents* (Philadelphia: Continental Company, 1904), vi–vii.

31. Ibid., 109.

32. Carolyn Conan Van Blarcom, *Getting Ready to Be a Mother: Information and Advice for the Young Woman who is Looking Forward to Motherhood* (New York: The Macmillan Company, 1937).

33. Ibid., 13.

34. Eastman, *Expectant Motherhood,* 75.

35. Ibid., 77.

36. The Boston Children's Medical Center, *Pregnancy, Birth & The Newborn Baby: A Publication for Parents* (Boston: Delacorte Press, 1972), 10.

37. Sylvia Smeal, *Unlike the Elephant* (London: Astra Books, 1951), 18, 29.

38. Ibid., 33.

39. Scott Mactavish, *The New Dad's Survival Guide: Man-to-Man Advice for First-Time Fathers* (New York: Little, Brown and Company, 2005).

40. Sullivan, S. Adams, *The Father's Almanac: From Pregnancy to Pre-School, Baby Care to Behavior, the Complete and Indispensable Book of Practical Advice and Ideas for Every Man Discovering the Fun and Challenge of Fatherhood* (New York: Bantam Doubleday, 1992).

41. Ian Davis, *My Boys Can Swim: The Official Guy's Guide to Pregnancy* (New York: Prima Publishing, 1999).

42. Dorrie Williams-Wheeler, *The Unplanned Pregnancy Book for Teens and College Students* (Virginia Beach: Sparkledoll Productions Publishing, 2004).

43. Denise Austin, *Denise Austin's Ultimate Pregnancy Book* (New York: Simon & Schuster, Inc. 1999).

44. Brooke Shields, *Down Came the Rain: My Journey Through Postpartum Depression* (New York: Hyperion Press, 2005).

45. Jenny McCarthy, *Belly Laughs: The Naked Truth about Pregnancy and Childbirth* (Cambridge, MA: Perseus Books, 2006).

46. Vicki Iovine, *The Girlfriends' Guide to Pregnancy* (New York: Pocket Books, 1999).

47. Ibid., xviii.

48. Babycenter.com Discussion Board, http://www.babycenter.com/ (accessed March 16, 2004).

49. Abby, Interview.

50. Frances, Interview.

51. Abby, Interview.

52. Beth, Interview.

53. Babycenter.com discussion board, http://www.babycenter.com/memberben efits/index.htm?v=pregnancy_mag&scid=GOO:SiteBrand:BabyCenterBrand&ef_id =SvQVcENIYWUAAERZDIcAAAAA:20120625210244:s (accessed March 18, 2004).

54. Ibid.

55. Abby, Interview.

56. Ibid.

57. Hoffert, *Private Matters,* 143.

58. Babycenter.com discussion board (accessed March 18, 2004).

59. Ibid.

60. Ibid.

61. Abby, interview.

62. Lauri Umansky, *Motherhood Reconceived: Feminism and the Legacies of the Sixties* (New York: New York University Press, 1996), 65.

63. They were interviewed on the program on August 29, 2006.

64. "The Gestation Project," www.enjoyyourdigitallife.com (accessed September 21, 2006).

65. Steven Zeitchik, "B&N Nurtures Pregnancy Book," *Publishers Weekly* 251, no. 50 (December 13, 2004), 10.

Chapter 4 A Pregnant Pause

1. Milt Josefsberg and Ben Starr, "Gloria is Nervous," *All in the Family*, season 6, episode 13, directed by Paul Bogart, aired December 8, 1975 (CBS).

2. Spar, *The Baby Business*, 7.

3. Anita Diamant, *The Red Tent* (New York: Picador USA, 1997).

4. Mazzoni, *Maternal Impressions*, 18.

5. Jessica Oppenheimer, Madelyn Davis, and Bob Carroll Jr., "Lucy is Enceinte," *I Love Lucy*, season 2, episode 10, directed by William Asher, aired December 8, 1952 (CBS).

6. Norman Lear, Johnny Speight, and Hal Kanter, "The Very Moving Day," *All in the Family*, season 6, episode 1, directed by Paul Bogart, aired September 8, 1975 (CBS).

7. Richard Baer and Sol Saks, "Alias Darrin Stephens," *Bewitched*, season 2, episode 2, directed by William Asher, aired September 16, 1965 (ABC).

8. Jeff Franklin and Boyd Hale, "Rock the Cradle," *Full House*, season 4, episode 26, directed by Joel Zwick, aired May 3, 1991 (ABC).

9. David Crane, Marta Kauffman, and Scott Silveri, "The One With Phoebe's Birthday Dinner," *Friends*, season 9, episode 5, directed by David Schwimmer, aired October 31, 2002 (NBC).

10. Liberty Godshall and Ann Lewis Hamilton, "Love and Sex," *Thirtysomething*, season 3, episode 2, directed by Marshall Herskovitz, aired October 3, 1989 (ABC).

11. Michael J. Weithorn, "Walk, Man," *King of Queens*, season 4, episode 1, directed by Rob Schiller, aired September 24, 2001 (CBS).

12. Richard J. Feinstein, "Ovary Action," *King of Queens*, season 4, episode 12, directed by Rob Schiller, aired December 17, 2001 (CBS).

13. Carter Bays and Craig Thomas, "Big Days," *How I Met Your Mother*, season 6, episode 1, directed by Pamela Fryman, aired September 20, 2010 (CBS).

14. *Notes from the Underbelly*, season 1, 2007 (ABC).

15. Abraham Higginbotham and Dan O'Shannon, "Aunt Mommy," *Modern Family*, season 3, episode 15, directed by Michael Spiller, aired February 15, 2012 (ABC).

16. Michael McCullers, *Baby Mama,* directed by Michael McCullers (Universal City, CA: Universal 2008).

17. Kate Angelo, *The Back-Up Plan,* directed by Alan Poul (Los Angeles, CA.: CBS Films, 2010).

18. Allan Loeb and Jeffrey Eugenides, *The Switch,* directed by Josh Gordon and Will Speck (Santa Monica, CA: Miramax, 2010).

19. Website of tvfanatic.com, http://www.tvfanatic.com/. Conception, once a taboo discussion for programs, is now public fodder for social media.

20. Amber Dowling, "Pregnancy ruins good TV," TVguide.ca, http://tvguide.ca/home/ (accessed April, 2007).

21. Jon Robin Baitz and Jessica Mecklenburg, "For the Children," *Brothers and Sisters,* season 1, episode 6, directed by Frederick E. O. Toye, aired October 29, 2006 (ABC).

22. Patrick Braoudé and Chris Columbus, *Nine Months,* directed by Chris Columbus (Century City, CA: 20th Century Fox, 1995).

23. Judd Apatow, *Knocked up,* directed by Judd Apatow (Universal City, CA: Universal, 2007).

24. Tony Kushner and Eric Roth, *Munich,* directed by Steven Spielberg (Universal City, CA: Universal, 2005).

25. Adrienne Shelly, *Waitress,* directed by Adrienne Shelly (Century City, CA, Fox Searchlight, 2007).

26. "Too Shaky for the Baby," *Tori & Dean,* directed by Robert Sizemore, season 1, episode 2, aired May 27, 2007 (Oxygen).

27. *Scott Baio is 46 . . . and Pregnant,* season 2, 2008, directed by Rich Kim (VH1).

28. Darren Star, "Beach Blanket Brandon," *Beverly Hills 90210,* season 2, episode 1, directed by Charles Braverman, aired July 11, 1991 (FOX).

29. Brenda Hampton, "Falling in Love," *The Secret Life of the American Teenager,* season 1, episode 1, directed by Ron Underwood, aired September 3, 2008 (ABC Family).

30. Meredith Blake, "Tina Fey Shows Off the 'Larva Monster' Growing Inside Her," About (Late) Last Night, *LA Times,* April 20, 2011, http://latimesblogs.latimes.com/showtracker/2011/04/about-late-last-night-tina-fey-shows-off-the-larva-monster-growing-inside-of-her.html.

31. The third pregnancy involved the character of Phoebe serving as a surrogate for her brother and sister-in-law.

32. David Crane and Marta Kauffman, "The One with the Sonogram at the End," *Friends,* season 1 episode 2, directed by James Burrows, aired September 29, 1994 (NBC).

33. Sherry Bilsing-Graham and Ellen Plummer, "The One Where Rachel Tells," *Friends,* season 8, episode 3, directed by Sheldon Epps, aired October 11, 2011 (NBC).

34. Brenda Hampton, "It Takes Two, Baby," *7th Heaven,* season 3, episode 1, directed by Burt Brinckerhoff, aired September 21, 1998 (WB).

35. Braoudé and Columbus, *Nine Months.*

36. Cody Diablo, *Juno,* directed by Jason Reitman (Century City, CA: Fox Searchlight, 2007).

37. Taylor, "A Fetish Is Born."

38. Laura Tropp, "Faking a Sonogram: Representations of Motherhood on Sex and the City," *Journal of Popular Culture* 39, no. 5 (2006), 861–877.

39. Hugo Rifkind, "Brad Pitt and Angelina Joli in London Yesterday," *Times (London),* January 26, 2011, accessed Newspaper Source, Access no. 7EH1515724538.

40. Hanson, *A Cultural History of Pregnancy,* 13.

41. Dan O'Bannon, *Alien,* directed by Ridley Scott (Century City, CA: 20th Century Fox, 1979).

42. John Cobbs, "*Alien* as an Abortion Parable," *Literature Film Quarterly* 18, no. 3 (1990), 198–201.

43. Ira Levin and Roman Polanski, *Rosemary's Baby,* directed by Roman Polanski (Los Angeles, CA: Paramount Pictures, 1968).

44. David Lynch, *Eraserhead,* directed by David Lynch (American Film Institute: Los Angeles, CA. 1977).

45. Risk taking among pregnant women is a popular trend on television as *In Plain Sight* and *Missing;* both series with women in dangerous occupations find themselves pregnant.

46. *Alias,* season 5, 2005–2006 (ABC).

47. Mary Kate Goodwin-Kelly also explores fear and anxiety concerning pregnant women in the film *Fargo.* Mary Kate Goodwin-Kelly, "Pregnant Body and/ As Smoking Gun," *Motherhood Misconceived,* eds., Heather Addison, Mary Kate Goodwin-Kelly, and Elaine Roth (Albany, NY: State University of New York Press, 2009), 25.

48. Alfonso Cuarón, Timothy J. Sexton, David Arata, Mark Fergus, and Hawk Ostby, *Children of Men,* directed by Alfonso Cuarón (Los Angeles, CA: Universal, 2006).

49. Peter Schink and Scott Charles Stewart, *Legion,* directed by Scott Charles Stewart (Culver City, CA: Screen Gems, 2009).

50. Steven Philip Kramer, "Mind the Baby Gap," *New York Times,* Op-ed, April 18, 2012, http://www.nytimes.com/2012/04/19/opinion/mind-the-baby-gap.html.

51. Claude Binyon and Robert G. Kane, *Kisses for My President,* directed by Curtis Bernhardt (Burbank, CA: Warner Bros., 1964).

52. John Hughes, *She's Having a Baby,* directed by John Hughes (Hollywood, CA: Paramount Pictures, 1988).

53. Lowell Ganz and Babaloo Mandel, *Parenthood,* directed by Ron Howard (Los Angeles, CA: Universal, 1989). This popular film inspired two television programs. The first premiered in 1990 for one season. The second version premiered in 2010 and is currently still on the air.

54. Katherine Reback, *Fools Rush In,* directed by Andy Tennant (Culver City, CA: Columbia Pictures, 1997).

55. Jeffrey Price, Peter S. Seaman, Chris Miller, and Aron Warner, *Shrek the Third,* directed by Chris Miller and Raman Hui (Hollywood, CA: Paramount Pictures, 2007).

56. Shauna Cross and Heather Hach, *What to Expect When You're Expecting,* directed by Kirk Jones (Santa Monica, CA: Lionsgate, 2012).

57. Dave Eggers and Vendela Vida, *Away We Go,* directed by Sam Mendes (Universal City, CA: Focus Features, 2009).

58. Jennifer Westfeldt, *Friends with Kids,* directed by Jennifer Westfeldt (Los Angeles, CA: Roadside Attractions, 2011).

59. Arlie Russell Hochschild, *The Second Shift* (New York: Penguin Books, 2003).

60. One scholar, Judy Kutulas, has suggested that extraordinary births in cabs, elevators, or other public places serve to depict women as "maternity amazons" who are able to look calm while the men around them are losing their cool. See Judy Kutulas, "'Do I Look Like a Chick'?: Men, women, and Babies on Sitcom Maternity Stories," *American Studies* 39, no. 2 (Summer 1998), 23.

61. Tim Brooks and Earle Marsh, eds., "Mary Kay and Johnny," in *The Complete Directory to Prime Time Network and Cable TV Shows 1946-Present,* 6th ed. (New York: Ballantine Books, 1995), 651.

62. Frazier Moore, "50 Years Later, Mary Kay and Johnny Recall TV's First Sitcom," *The Columbia,* November 17, 1997, B7.

63. Carl Reiner, "Where did I come From?" *The Dick Van Dyke Show,* season 1, episode 19, directed by John Rich, aired January 3, 1962 (CBS).

64. Bernard Slade, "And Then There Were Three," *Bewitched,* season 2, episode 18, directed by William Asher, aired January 13, 1966 (ABC).

65. Cassidy, *Birth: The Surprising History,* 207.

66. Lou Derman and Milt Josefsberg, "Mike's Pains," *All in the Family,* season 6, episode 5, directed by Paul Bogart, aired October 6, 1975 (CBS).

67. Josefsberg and Starr, "Gloria is Nervous."

68. Lou Derman, Bill Davenport, Milt Josefsberg, Larry Rhine, Ben Starr, and Mel Tolkin, "Births of the Baby (Parts 1 & 2)," *All in the Family,* season 6, episodes 14 and 15, directed by Paul Bogart, aired December 15 and 22, 1975 (CBS).

69. Jeff Greenstein and Jeff Strauss, "The One with the Birth," *Friends,* season 1, episode 23, directed by James Burrows, aired May 11, 1995 (NBC).

70. Larry Charles, "The Birth (Parts 1 & 2)," *Mad about You,* season 5, episodes 23 and 24, directed by Gordon Hunt, aired May 20, 1997 (NBC).

71. Ann Lewis Hamilton, "New Baby," *Thirtysomething,* season 3, episode 4, directed by Marshall Herskovitz, aired October 24, 1989 (ABC).

72. Albert Hackett, Frances Goodrich, Nancy Meyers, and Charles Shyer, *Father of the Bride Part II,* directed by Charles Shyer (Burbank, CA: Buena Vista, 1995).

73. Brenda Hampton and Jeffrey Rodgers, "Paper or Plastic," *7th Heaven,* season 9, episode 12, directed by Michael Preece, aired January 24, 2005 (WB).

74. Jennifer Hendriks, "The Magician's Code: Part 1," *How I Met Your Mother,* season 7, episode 23, directed by Pamela Fryman, aired May 14, 2012 (CBS).

75. Gary Murphy, "Julie and Eric's Baby," *Notes from the Underbelly,* season 1, episode 5, directed by Barry Sonnenfeld, aired May 2, 2007 (ABC).

76. Caroline Williams, "Birth," *Up All Night,* season 1, episode 6, directed by Randall Einhorn, aired October 19, 2011 (NBC).

77. For more information about how television supports the dominant ideology that the medical establishment of doctors and hospitals are the best place to give birth, read Kimberly Kline's study of popular representation of midwives on television, where the midwives are made to look controlling and depicted as an irrational choice. Kimberly Kline, "Midwife Attended Births in Prime-Time Television: Craziness, Controlling Bitches, and Ultimate Capitulation," *Women & Language* 30, no. 1 (Spring 2007): 20–29.

78. Neil Genzingler, "Painful Baby Boom on Primetime TV," *New York Times,* November 2, 2011, http://www.nytimes.com/2011/11/03/arts/television/harrowing-births-on-prime-time-tv.html?pagewanted=all.

79. Jason Katims, "Nora," *Parenthood,* directed by Allison Liddi-Brown, season 3, episode 5, aired October 11, 2011 (NBC).

80. Jude Davies and Carol R. Smith, "Race, Gender, and the American Mother: Political Speech and the Maternity Episodes of *I Love Lucy* and *Murphy Brown*," *American Studies* 39, no. 2 (Summer 1998): 38.

Chapter 5 The Backseat Pregnancy

1. Cassidy, *Birth: The Surprising History,* 210.

2. Richard K. Reed, *Birthing Fathers: The Transformation of Men in American Rites of Birth* (New Brunswick, NJ: Rutgers University Press, 2005). Reed traces the history of men's involvement in birth and also explores cultures today where it is still practiced.

3. Shari Thurer, *The Myths of Motherhood: How Culture Reinvents the Good Mother* (New York: Penguin Books, 1994), 13.

4. Thurer, *The Myths of Motherhood,* 35.

5. Ibid., 62.

6. Sukanta Saha et al., "Advanced Paternal Age Is Associated with Impaired Neurocognitive Outcomes during Infancy and Childhood," *PLoS Med* 6, no. 3 (2009): e1000040. doi:10.1371/journal.pmed.10000.

7. Harry Fisch, *The Male Biological Clock: The Startling News about Aging, Sexuality, and Fertility in Men* (New York: Free Press, 2005).

8. Amelia Thomson-DeVeaux, "Guys' biological clocks are ticking too?" *Equal Writes,* April 7, 2009, http://equalwrites.org/2009/04/07/guys-biological-clocks-are-ticking-too/.

9. "The Biological Clock," New Hope Fertility Center, http://72.47.206.49/biological-clock.shtml (accessed September 10, 2010).

10. Spar, *The Baby Business,* 12.

11. Roberto Zapperi, *The Pregnant Man* (Chur, Switzerland; New York: Harwood Academic Publishers, 1991), 111. This book has an exhaustive history of images of male pregnancy from the Old Testament through more modern fables.

12. Zapperi, *The Pregnant Man,* 50, 93–95.

13. Catherine Orenstein, *Little Red Riding Hood Uncloaked: Sex, Morality, and the Evolution of a Fairy Tale* (New York: Basic Books, 2002), 194–95.

14. Howard Leeds, "A Very Special Delivery," *Bewitched,* season 2, episode 2, directed by William Asheraired on September 23, 1965 (ABC).

15. Jacques Demy, *A Slightly Pregnant Man* (L'événement le plus important depuis que l'homme a marché sur la lune), directed by Jacques Demy (France: Lira Films, 1973).

16. Joan Rivers and Jay Redack, *Rabbit Test,* directed by Joan Rivers (Culver City, CA: AVCO Embassy Pictures, 1978).

17. Carmen Finestra, Gary Kott, and John Markus, "The Day the Spores Landed," *The Cosby Show,* season 6, episode 8, directed by Neema Barnette, aired November 9, 1989 (NBC).

18. *The View,* season 12, episode 195, aired June 11, 2009 (ABC).

19. *Mario Lopez: Saved by the Baby,* season 1, 2010, directed by Clay Westervelt (VH1).

20. Alan R. Cohen, Alan Freedland, Adam Sztykiel and Todd Phillips, *Due Date,* directed by Todd Phillips (Burbank, CA: Warner Bros., 2010).

21. Rich Juzwiak, VH1Blog, log. http://blog.vh1.com/2010–05–31/examining-vh1-dad-camp-with-dr-jeff-episode-1 (accessed April 10, 2012).

22. Sarah Blaffer Hrdy, *Mother Nature: A History of Mothers, Infants, and Natural Selection* (New York: Pantheon, 1999), 217. This book provides a fascinating history of the evolution of motherhood and fatherhood in primates and then humans.

23. Hrdy, *Mother Nature,* 213–14.

24. Reed, *Birthing Fathers,* 40.

25. See Leavitt's book to read actual quotes from these journal notebooks from men who recorded their nervousness or even their gender preference (often a boy). Sarah A. Leavitt and Judith Walzer, *Make Room for Daddy: The Journey from Waiting Room to Birthing Room* (Chapel Hill: The University of North Carolina Press, 2009), 76.

26. Leavitt and Walzer, *Make Room for Daddy,* 100–101.

27. Ibid., 142.

28. Ibid., 251.

29. Shira Segal, "Homebirth Advocacy on the Internet," *Rupkatha Journal on Interdisciplinary Studies in Humanities* 2, 1 (2010), http://www.rupkatha.com/homebirthvdvocacy.php.

30. Jeremy Adam Smith, *The Daddy Shift. How Stay-at-Home Dads, Breadwinning Moms, and Shared Parenting are Transforming the American Family* (Boston: Beacon Press, 2009).

31. Louann Brizendine, *The Female Brain* (New York: Morgan Road Books, 2006), 104.

32. J. T. Condon and Boyce P. Corkindale, "The First-Time Fathers Study: A Prospective Study of the Mental Health and Well-Being of Men During the Transition to Parenthood," *Australian and New Zealand Journal of Psychiatry* 38, nos. 1–2 (January–February 2004): 56–64.

33. Orenstein, *Little Red Riding Hood Uncloaked,* 197.

Chapter 6 The Pregnancy Industrial Complex

1. Heide Murkoff, Arlene Eisenberg and Sandee Hathaway, *What to Expect When You're Expecting* (New York: Workman Publishing, 2002).

2. Moore, "50 Years Later," B7.

3. Davies and Smith, "Race, Gender, and the American Mother," 33–63.

4. "Mother Mill," *People Weekly,* May 5, 1974, 42.

5. "Star Tracks," *People Weekly,* July 29, 1974, 24.

6. "The Rick Nelsons Come of Age," *People Weekly,* May 27, 1974, 42.

7. "Medics," *People Weekly,* June 10, 1974, 33.

8. *People Weekly,* September 23, 1974, 13.

9. "Medics," *People Weekly,* June 10, 1974, 33.

10. "Lookout," *People Weekly,* June 3, 1974, 35.

11. "Star Tracks," *People Weekly,* June 10, 1974, 24, 19.

12. Dave Karger, "Angelina Jolie: A Candid Q&A," *EW.com Entertainment Weekly,* June 11, 2008, http://www.ew.com/ew/article/0,,20205854,00.html.

13. "World Exclusive: Matthew & Camila's Baby Boy," *OK Magazine,* July 23, 2008, http://www.okmagazine.com/babies/world-exclusive-matthew-camilas-baby-boy.

14. Susan J. Douglas and Meredith W. Michaels, *The Mommy Myth: The Idealization of Motherhood and How It Has Undermined Women* (New York: Free Press, 2004), 4–5.

15. Jon Caramanica, "Night of Validation for Young Stars (and Censors)," *New York Times,* August 30, 2011, late edition, C3.

16. Nina Bernstein, "After Beyoncé Gives Birth, Patients Protest Celebrity Security at Lenox Hill Hospital," *New York Times,* January 9, 2012, http://www.nytimes.com/2012/01/10/nyregion/after-birth-by-beyonce-patients-protest-celebrity-security-at-lenox-hill-hospital.html.

17. "Mailbag," *People Weekly,* August 18, 2003, 4.

18. Gélis, *History of Childbirth,* 80.

19. Carter and Duriez, *With Child: Birth,* 45.

20. Bull, *Hints to Mothers,* 32.

21. Hoffert, *Private Matters,* 31–32.

22. Ibid., 31.

23. Van Blarcom, *Getting Ready to Be a Mother,* 23.

24. Richard W. Wertz and Dorothy C. Wertz, *Lying-In: A History of Childbirth in America* (New York: Free Press, 1977).

25. Web Site of Destination Maternity Corporation, http://heidiklum.destinationmaternity.com.

26. Ruth La Ferla, "Showing? It's Time to Show Off," *New York Times,* June 8, 2006, G1.

27. Sara Libby, "Is Forever 21 Glamorizing Teen Pregnancy?" *Salon,* July 20, 2010, http://www.salon.com/2010/07/20/forever_21_maternity/.

28. "Maternity Tees," *People,* July 12, 2006.

29. La Ferla, "Showing? It's Time," G1.

30. Mireya Navaroo, "Here Comes the Mother-to-Be," *New York Times,* March 13, 2005, section 9, 1.

31. Sandra Matthews and Laura Wexler provide a fascinating history of the evolution of pregnancy photography: Sandra Matthews and Laura Wexler, *Pregnant Pictures* (New York: Routledge, 2000).

32. Anju Mary Paul, "Pregnant Bellies Auctioned as Ad Space on eBay," *Women's eNews,* March 19, 2006, http://womensenews.org/story/business/060319/pregnant-bellies-auctioned-ad-space-ebay (accessed January 23, 2010).

33. Eckard, *Maternal Body and Voice,* 23.

34. Marisa Belger, "Beyond Bliss: Inside NYC's Only Organic Spa," *TODAY.com,* January 7, 2008, http://today.msnbc.msn.com/id/22544570/ns/today-green/t/beyond-bliss-inside-nycs-only-organic-spa/#.T-gzB_XNmPM (accessed January 23, 2010).

35. Stonyfield Farm, "Stonyfield Farm Introduces First Yogurt for Expectant, Nursing, and New Moms and Beyond," press release January 18, 2008, http://www.prlog.org/10046450-stonyfield-farm-introduces-first-yogurt-for-expectant-nursing-and-new-moms-and-beyond.html.

36. Kao USA (Curel), http://www.curel.com/pregnancy (accessed January 2010).

37. *New York Magazine,* "Best Baby Gear Guru," Best of New York, 2010, www.nymag.com/bestofny/kids/2010/baby-gear/.

38. Ellie and Melissa, The Baby Planners, http://www.thebabyplanners.com

39. Arlie Russell Hochschild, *The Outsourced Life: Intimate Life in Market Times* (New York: Metropolitan Books, 2012), 223.

40. "Jennifer Lopez's Baby Shower," *AskMen.Com Newsletter,* January 18, 2008, http://www.askmen.com/celebs/entertainment-news/jennifer-lopez/jennifer-lopezs-baby-shower.html.

41. Plan the Perfect Baby Shower, http://www.plan-the-perfect-baby-shower.com/celebrity-baby-showers.html.

42. Alex Williams and Kate Murphy, "A Boy or Girl? Cut the Cake," *New York Times,* April 8, 2012, 1–2.

43. "What about This Offer?" Starwood Hotels & Resorts Worldwide, http://www.starwoodpromos.com/whotelsbabyme/ (accessed June 25, 2012).

44. "Deals From Marriott," Marriott International, http://www.marriott.com/specials/mesOffer.mi?marrOfferId=159449 (accessed January 12, 2010).

45. For an interesting discussion of the evolution of the parenting expert and the public's reliance on them, read Pamela Paul, *Parenting, Inc.*

Chapter 7 Womb Time

1. *Pregnant in Heels,* season1 and 2, 2011 and 2012 (Bravo).

2. "Clueless," *Pregnant in Heels,* season 1, episode 4, aired April 26, 2011 (Bravo).

3. Ibid.

4. The couple ended up choosing the name Bowen, against the recommendations of the consultants and focus groups.

5. "Homebirth with a Side of Placenta," *Pregnant in Heels,* season 2, episode 1, May 15, 2012 (Bravo).

6. Ken Levine, "Bravo's Pregnant in Heels—Oh My Fucking God!, *The World as Seen by a TV Comedy Writer* (Blog), April 6, 2011, http://kenlevine.blogspot.com/2011/04/bravos-pregnant-in-heels-oh-my-fucking.html (accessed May 30, 2012).

7. *Tia & Tamara,* season 1 and 2, 2011 and 2012 (Style Network).

8. "Acting the Part," *Tia & Tamara,* season 1, episode 6, September 19, 2011 (Style).

9. Jacob Bernstein, "The Baby Bump," *New York Times,* April 29, 2012, styles section.

10. Jeanine Poggi, "As 'Jersey Shore' Drifts, MTV promotes pregnant Snooki," *Ad Age,* April 27, 2012, http://adage.com/article/special-report-tv-upfront/jersey-shore-drifts-mtv-promotes-pregnant-snooki/234423/.

11. Neil Postman, *Amusing Ourselves to Death: Public Discourse in the Age of Show Business* (New York: Penguin Books, 1985).

12. Jo Casamento, "Oh Baby, That's a Lot of Money; THE Goss," *Sun Herald (Sydney),* May 27, 2012, LexisNexis Academic.

13. Camilla Long, "Bumponomics," *Sunday Times (London),* May 13, 2012, style section, LexisNexis Academic.

14. The company filed for bankruptcy in 2011. Maria Panaritis, "Children's Clothier Hartstrings Declares Bankruptcy," *Philadelphia Inquirer,* June 4, 2011, A07.

15. Thurer, *The Myths of Motherhood,* 233.

16. Andrew Adam Newman, "Maker of Pregnancy Test Finds Opportunity in Personal Stories," *New York Times,* May 2, 2010, http://www.nytimes.com/2010/05/03/business/media/03adco.html.

17. Elissa Gootman, "So Eager for Grandchildren, They're Paying the Egg-Freezing Clinic," *New York Times,* May 13, 2012.

18. Jolie O'Dell, "Facebook adds Pregnancy Profile option: Let the Ads Begin!" *VentureBeat,* August 1, 2011, http://venturebeat.com/2011/08/01/facebook-pregnant/.

19. Nat Ives, "American Baby Customizes Issues for Subscribers' Stage of Pregnancy or Motherhood," *Ad Age Media News,* September 29, 2001, http://adage.com/article/media/american-baby-customizes-issues-stages-pregnancy/230106/.

20. Neil Howe and William Strauss, *Millennials Rising: The Next Great Generation* (New York: Vintage Books, 2000).

21. Nattavudh Powdthavee, "Think Having Children Will Make You Happy?" *The Psychologist, Online Journal of the British Psychological Society* 22, part 4 (April 2009), http://www.thepsychologist.org.uk/archive/archive_home.cfm?volumeID=22&editionID=174&ArticleID=1493.

22. Charles Duhigg, "How Companies Learn Your Secrets," *New York Times Magazine,* February 16, 2012, http://www.nytimes.com/2012/02/19/magazine/shopping-habits.html?pagewanted=all.

23. *I'm pregnant and …,* seasons 1 and 2, 2009–2011 (Discovery Health).

24. *I Didn't Know I was Pregnant,* seasons 1–4, 2008–2011 (TLC).

25. *Sixteen and Pregnant,* seasons 1–5, 2009–2012 (MTV).

26. James Dinh, "MTV's 16 and Pregnant Credited for Decline in Teen Pregnancy Rates," *MTV Network,* December 22, 2010, http://www.mtv.com/news/articles/1654818/mtvs-16-pregnant-credited-decline-teen-pregnancy-rates.jhtml.

27. "Jennifer," *Sixteen and Pregnant,* season 3, episode 2, aired July 23, 2009 (MTV).

28. Paul, *Origins: How the Nine Months,* 70.

29. Eve Tahmincioglue, "Pregnant Workers Filing More Complaints of Bias," *New York Times,* September 14, 2003, section 10. These increases may actually be higher because many cases do not actually reach the federal level where they are reported.

30. Noreen Farrell, Jamie Dolkas, and Mia Munro, "Expecting A Baby, Not A Lay-Off: Why Federal Law Should Require The Reasonable Accommodation of Pregnant Workers," Report Prepared by the Equal Rights Advocates, May 10, 2012, http://www.equalrights.org/media/2012/ERA-PregAccomReport.pdf.

31. Associated Press, "Commander to Rescind a Provision on Pregnancy," *New York Times,* December 25, 2009.

32. Amy Joyce, "Pregnancy Case Yields Payout of $48.9 million," *Washington Post,* June 6, 2006.

33. Warren Richey, "Old Maternity Leave Won't Count toward Pensions," *Christian Science Monitor,* May 18, 2009.

34. David W. Chen, "Discrimination Suit against Bloomberg L.P. is Rejected," *New York Times,* August 17, 2011.

35. KJ Dell'Antonia, "Protection for Pregnant Workers," Motherlode (blog), *New York Times,* May 8, 2012, http://parenting.blogs.nytimes.com/2012/05/08/protection-for-pregnant-workers/.

36. Jack Mirkinson, "Megyn Kelly Demolishes Mike Gallagher for Calling Her Maternity Leave a 'Racket'," *Huffington Post,* August 9, 2011, last modified October 9, 2011, http://www.huffingtonpost.com/2011/08/09/megyn-kelly-mike-gallagher-maternity-leave_n_922393.html.

37. Mazzoni, *Maternal Impressions,* 6.

38. Annie Murphy Paul, "Too Fat and Pregnant: The Maternal Risks of Obesity," *New York Times,* July 13, 2008, 19.

39. Molly M. Ginty, "Female Troubles for Wildlife Raise Human Worries," *Women's eNews,* December 18, 2006, http://womensenews.org/story/environment/061218/female-troubles-wildlife-raise-human-worries.

40. Alex Kuczynski, "The Nine Months of Living Anxiously," *New York Times,* May 23, 2004, section 9.

41. Gina Kolata, "Pregnant Exercisers Test Limits," *New York Times,* November 8, 2007, G1, G8.

42. Lourdes Garcia-Navarro, "It's A Boy: War Reporter's Baby Shower in Baghdad," *NPR's Morning Edition,* July 6, 2010, http://www.npr.org/templates/story/story.php?storyId=128061606NPR.org.

43. Shonda Rhimes and Stacy McKee, "What Have I Done to Deserve This?" *Grey's Anatomy,* season 2, episode 19, directed by Wendey Stanzler, aired on February 26, 2006 (NBC).

44. Tina Fey and Jack Burditt, "Jack Meets Dennis," *30 Rock,* season 1, episode 6, directed by Juan José Campanella, aired on November 30, 2006 (NBC).

45. William Safire, "Bump," On Language, *New York Times Magazine,* May 14, 2006. 22.

46. *Urban Dictionary,* September 2, 2008, http://www.urbandictionary.com / define.php?term=baby%20bump.

47. For a fascinating analysis of this type of advertising, read Janelle S. Taylor, "The Public Fetus and the Family Car: From Abortion Politics to a Volvo Advertisement," *Public Culture* 4, no. 2 (Spring 1992): 67–80.

48. David Kiley, "Carl's Jr. Fetus Ads Creepier than a Jr. High School Health Film," *Bloomberg Business Week,* April 11, 2005, http://www.businessweek.com/the_thread/brandnewday/archives/2005/04/carls_jr_fetus.html.

49. Brian Dakss, "Pregnant Woman Loses HOV Lane Case," CBS News, January 12, 2006, http://www.cbsnews.com/2100–500202_162–1203514.html.

50. Banerjee, "Church Groups Turn to Sonogram."

51. Amanda Marcotte, "Randall Terry's Self-Promoting Super Bowl Fetus Ads," *Guardian* (Manchester), January 12, 2012, http://www.guardian.co.uk/commentisfree/cifamerica /2012/jan/12/randall-terry-super-bowl-fetus-ads.

52. Adam Liptak, "Putting the Government's Words in the Doctor's Mouth," *New York Times,* August 6, 2007.

53. Kevin Sack, "In Ultrasound, Abortion Fight Has New Front," *New York Times,* May 28, 2010.

54. Erick Eckholm and Kim Severson, "Other States Take Notice of Measure on Abortion," *New York Times,* February 29, 2012, Academic Search Premier (Access no. 72085435).

55. Laury Oaks, "Smoke-Filled Wombs and Fragile Fetuses: The Social Politics of Fetal Representation," *Signs: Journal of Women in Culture and Society,* 26, no. 1 (2000), 63–108.

56. Ada Calhoun, "Mommy Had to go Away for A While," *New York Times Magazine,* April 29, 2012, MM30.

57. Oaks, "Smoke-Filled Wombs," 100.

58. Clara Totenberg Green, "Nebraska Laws Ban Abortions Based on Fetal Pain, Challenging 35 Years of Constitutionally Protected Reproductive Freedom," *Legal Momentum,* The Women's Legal Defense and Education Fund, April 20, 2010, http://legalmomentum.typepad.com/blog/2010/04/nebraska-laws-ban-abortions-based-on-fetal-pain-challenging-35-years-of-constitutionally-protected-r.html.

59. Annie Murphy Paul, "The First Ache," *New York Times Magazine,* February 10, 2008, 49.

60. Cara Litke, "Pregnant Chicks Who Brag Too Much," *Cosmopolitan,* http://www.cosmopolitan.com/advice/tips/pregnant-chicks-who-brag-too-much (accessed August 21, 2011).

61. Jen Doll, "Should You Get Special Privileges for Getting Knocked Up?" January 24, 2011, *The Village Voice Blogs,* http://blogs.villagevoice.com/runninscared/2011/01/should_you_get.php.

62. Thurer, *The Myths of Motherhood,* 105.

63. Ibid., 178.

64. Rickie Solinger, *Pregnancy and Power: A Short History of Reproductive Politics in America* (New York: New York University Press, 2005), 105.

65. Robbie Davis-Floyd, *Birth as an American Rite of Passage* (Los Angeles: University of California Press, 1992), 305.

Chapter 8 The Big Let-Down

1. Pregnancy-Info.net, http://www.pregnancy-info.net/.

2. Roni Caryn Rabin, "With New Test, Men Can Have At-Home Fertility Screening," *New York Times,* June 4, 2007, A12.

3. Pam Belluck, "Scientific Advances on Contraceptive for Men," *New York Times,* July 23, 2011.

4. For more information on the legal rights of fathers, see James M. Humber and Robert F. Almeder, eds., *Reproduction, Technology, and Rights* (Totowa, NJ: Humana Press, 1996).

5. Tina Cassidy, "Birth, Controlled," *New York Times,* March 26, 2006, http://www.nytimes.com/2006/03/26/magazine/326wwln_essay.html.

6. Jane E. Brody, "A Campaign to Carry Pregnancies to Term," *New York Times,* August 8, 2011, 8

7. U.S. Food and Drug Administration, "Radiation-Emitting Products," http://www.fda.gov/radiation-emittingproducts/default.htm (accessed July 7, 2007).

8. Claudia Kolker, *The Immigrant Advantage: What We Can Learn from Newcomers to America about Health, Happiness and Hope* (New York: Free Press, 2011), 38–61.

9. Shields, *Down Came the Rain,* 57–60.

10. "Gwyneth Paltrow and Bryce Dallas Howard Describe Postpartum Depression," *Huffington Post,* July 22, 2010, http://www.chicagomanualofstyle.org/16/ch14/ch14_sec200.html.

11. Laura Tropp, "Off Their Rockers: Representation of Postpartum Depression," *Mental Illness in Popular Media: Essays on the Representation of Disorders,* ed. Lawrence C. Rubin (Jefferson, NC: McFarland, 2012), 77–91.

12. Neil Postman, *Technopoly: The Surrender of Culture to Technology* (New York: Knopf, 1992).

Bibliography

"Acting the Part." *Tia and Tamara.* Season 1, episode 6, aired September 19, 2011 (Style Network).

Adams, Sullivan S. *The Father's Almanac: From Pregnancy to Pre-School, Baby Care to Behavior, the Complete and Indispensable Book of Practical Advice and Ideas for Every Man Discovering the Fun and Challenge of Fatherhood.* New York: Bantam Doubleday, 1992.

AdRants. n.d. AdRants, http://www.adrants.com/2004/10/pregnancy-test-suspense-sells-harlequin-b.php (accessed August 1, 2007).

Alias. Season 5, 2005–2006 (ABC).

"American Baby Customizes Issues for Subscribers' Stage of Pregnancy or Motherhood." *Ad Age Media News.* September 29, 2001. http://adage.com/article/media/american-baby-customizes-issues-stages-pregnancy/230106/.

American Pregnancy Association. *americanpregnancy.org.* n.d. http://www.american-pregnancy.org/.

Angelo, Kate. *The Back-Up Plan.* Directed by Alan Poul. Produced by CBS Films. Los Angeles, CA. 2010.

Apatow, Judd. *Knocked up.* Directed by Judd Apatow. Produced by Universal. Universal City, CA. 2007.

Associated Press. "Commander to Rescind a Provision on Pregnancy." *New York Times,* December 25, 2009.

Austin, Denise. *Denise Austin's Ultimate Pregnancy Book.* New York: Simon & Schuster, Inc., 1999.

Babble Boards: Pregnancy. n.d. http://www.babble.com/ (accessed July 17, 2007).

BabyCenter, L.L.C. *babycenter.com.* n.d. http://www.babycenter.com/.

Babyplus Company LLC, The. n.d. http://www.babyplus.com/.

Baer, Richard, and Sol Saks. "Alias Darrin Stephens." *Bewitched.* Season 2, episode 2, directed by William Asher, aired September 16, 1965 (ABC).

Baitz, Jon Robin, and Jessica Mecklenburg. "For the Children." *Brothers and Sisters.* Season 1, episode 6, directed by Frederick E.O. Toye, aired October 29, 2006 (ABC).

Banerjee, Neela. "Church Groups Turn to Sonogram to Turn Women from Abortions." *New York Times,* February 2, 2005: A1, A15.

Banerjee, Neela. "Church Groups Turn to Sonogram to Turn Women From Abortions." *New York Times,* February 2, 2005.

Bays, Carter, and Craig Thomas. "Big Days." *How I Met Your Mother.* Season 6, episode 1, directed by Pamela Fryman, aired September 20, 2010 (CBS).

Belger, Marisa. "Beyond Bliss: Inside NYC's Only Organic Spa." *TODAY.com.* January 7, 2008. http://today.msnbc.msn.com/id/22544570/ns/today-green/t/beyond-bliss-inside-nycs-only-organic-spa/#.T-gzB_XNmPM (accessed January 23, 2010).

Belluck, Pam. "Scientific Advances on Contraceptive for Men." *New York Times,* July 23, 2011.

Belluck, Pam. "Test Can Tell Fetal Sex at 7 Weeks, Study Says." *New York Times,* August 9, 2011.

Bernstein, Jacob. "The Baby Bump." *New York Times,* April 29, 2012: Styles.

Bernstein, Nina. "After Beyoncé Gives Birth, Patients Protest Celebrity Security at Lenox Hill Hospital." *New York Times,* January 9, 2012.

"Best Baby Gear Guru." *New York Magazine, Best of New York.* 2010. http://nymag.com/bestofny/kids/2010/baby-gear/.

Bilsing-Graham, Sherry, and Ellen Plummer. "The One Where Rachel Tells." *Friends.* Season 8, episode 3, directed by Sheldon Epps, aired October 11, 2011 (NBC).

Binyon, Claude, and Robert G. Kane. *Kisses for My President.* Directed by Curtis Bernhardt. Produced by Warner Bros. Burbank, CA. 1964.

Blake, Meredith. "Tina Fey Shows Off the 'Larva Monster' Growing Inside Her." *LA Times,* April 20, 2011. http://latimesblogs.latimes.com/showtracker/2011/04/about-late-last-night-tina-fey-shows-off-the-larva-monster-growing-inside-of-her.html.

Boston Children's Medical Center. *Pregnancy, Birth & The Newborn Baby: A Publication for Parents.* Boston: Delacorte Press, 1972.

Braoudé, Patrick, and Chris Columbus. *Nine Months.* Directed by Chris Columbus. Produced by 20th Century Fox. Century City, CA. 1995.

Brizendine, Jouann. *The Female Brain.* New York: Morgan Road Books, 2006.

Brooks, Tim, and Earle Marsh. *The Complete Directory to Prime Time Network and Cable TV Shows 1946-Present.* 6th. New York: Ballantine Books, 1995.

Bull, Thomas. *Hints to Mothers, for the Management of Health During the Period of Pregnancy, and in the Lying-In Room; with an Exposure of Popular Errors in Connexion with Those Subjects.* 3rd London edition (Reprinted in History of Women, New Haven, CT: Research Publications, Inc., 1975). New York: Wiley & Putnam, 1842.

BYG Publishing, Inc. *bygpub.com.* n.d. http://www.bygpub.com/natural/pregnancy.htm.

BYG Publishing, Inc. n.d. http://www.bygpub.com/natural/pregnancy.htm.

Calhoun, Ada. "Mommy Had to go Away for A While." *New York Times Magazine,* April 29, 2012: MM30.

Caramanica, Jon. "Night of Validation for Young Stars (and Censors)." *New York Times,* August 30, 2011.

Carter, Jenny, and Thérèse Duriez. *With Child: Birth Through the Ages.* Edinburgh: Mainstream Publishing, 1986.

Casamento, Jo. "Oh Baby, That's a Lot of Money; THE Goss." *Sun Herald (Sydney),* May 27, 2012.

Cassidy, Tina. *Birth: The Surprising History of How We are Born.* New York: Atlantic Monthly Press, 2006.

Cassidy, Tina. "Birth, Controlled." *New York Times,* March 26, 2006. http://www.nytimes.com/2006/03/26/magazine/326wwln_essay.html.

Charles, Larry. "The Birth (Parts 1 & 2)." *Mad About You.* Season 5, episodes 23 and 24, aired May 20, 1997 (NBC).

Chavasee, Pye Henry. *Advice to a Mother on the Management of Her Children: And on the Treatment on the Moment of Some of Their More Pressing Illnesses and Accidents.* Philadelphia: Continental Company, 1904.

Chen, David W. "Discrimination Suit Against Bloomberg L.P. is Rejected." *New York Times,* August 17, 2011.

Church & Dwight Co., Inc. *First Response Website.* n.d. http://www.firstresponse.com/index.asp (accessed August 1, 2007).

"Clueless." *Pregnant in Heels.* Season 1, episode 4, aired April 26, 2011 (Bravo).

Cobbs, John. "Alien as an Abortion Parable." *Literature Film Quarterly* 18, no. 3 (1990): 198–201.

Cohen, Alan R., Alan Freedland, Adam Sztykiel, and Todd Phillips. *Due Date.* Directed by Todd Phillips. Produced by Warner Bros., Burbank, CA. 2010.

Condon, J.T., and Boyce P. Corkindale. "The First-Time Fathers Study: A Prospective Study of the Mental Health and Well-Being of Men During the Transition to Parenthood." *Australian and New Zealand Journal of Psychiatry* 38, no. 1–2 (Jan-Feb 2004): 56–64.

Crane, David, and Marta Kauffman. "The One with the Sonogram at the End." *Friends.* Season 1 episode 2, directed by James Burrows, aired September 29, 1994 (NBC).

Crane, David, Marta Kauffman, and Scott Silveri. "The One With Phoebe's Birthday Dinner." *Friends.* Season 9, episode 5, directed by David Schwimmer, aired October 31, 2002 (NBC).

Cross, Shauna, and Heather Hach. *What to Expect When You're Expecting.* Directed by Kirk Jones. Produced by Lionsgate. Santa Monica, CA. 2012.

Cuarón, Alfonso, Timothy J. Sexton, David Arata, Mark Fergus, and Hawk Ostby. *Children of Men.* Directed by Alfonso Cuarón. Produced by Universal. Los Angeles, CA. 2006.

Curtis, Michael. "The One with the Princess Leia Fantasy." *Friends.* Season 3, episode 1, directed by Gail Mancuso,(FOX), aired September 19, 1996.

Dakss, Brian. "Pregnant Woman Loses HOV Lane Case," CBS News." *CBS News.* January 12, 2012. http://www.cbsnews.com/2100–500202_162–1203514.html.

Davies, Jude, and Carol R. Smith. "Race, Gender, and the American Mother: Political Speech and the Maternity Episodes of I Love Lucy and Murphy Brown." *American Studies* 39, no. 2 (Summer 1998): 33–63.

Davis, Ian. *My Boys Can Swim: The Official Guy's Guide to Pregnancy.* New York: Prima Publishing, 1999.

Davis-Floyd, Robbie. *Birth as an American Rite of Passage.* Los Angeles: University of California Press, 1992.

"Deals from Marriott." *Marriott International.* n.d. http://www.marriott.com/ specials/mesOffer.mi?marrOfferId=159449 (accessed January 12, 2010).

Dell'Antonia, K. J. "Protection for Pregnant Workers." *Motherlode (blog), New York Times,* May 8, 2012. http://parenting.blogs.nytimes.com/2012/05/08/protection-for-pregnant-workers/.

Demy, Jacques. *A Slightly Pregnant Man (L'événement le plus important depuis que l'homme a marché sur la lune).* Directed by Jacques Demy. Produced by Lira Films, France. 1973.

Derman, Lou, and Milt Josefsberg. "Mike's Pains." *All in the Family.* Season 6, episode 5, directed by Paul Bogart, aired October 6, 1975 (CBS).

Derman, Lou, Bill Davenport, Milt Josefsberg, Larry Rhine, Ben Starr, and Mel Tolkin. "Births of the Baby (Parts 1 & 2)." *All in the Family.* Season 6, episodes 14 and 15, directed by Paul Bogart, aired December 15 and 22, 1975 (CBS).

Destination Maternity Corporation. n.d. http://heidiklum.destinationmaternity.com.

Diablo, Cody. *Juno.* Directed by Jason Reitman. Produced by Fox Searchlight. Century City, CA. 2007.

Diamant, Anita. *The Red Tent.* New York: Picador USA, 1997.

Dinh, James. "MTV's 16 and Pregnant Credited for Decline in Teen Pregnancy Rates." *MTV Network.* December 22, 2010. http://www.mtv.com/news/articles/1654818/mtvs-16-pregnant-credited-decline-teen-pregnancy-rates.jhtml.

Doll, Jen. "Should You Get Special Privileges for Getting Knocked Up?" *The Village Voice Blogs.* January 24, 2011. http://blogs.villagevoice.com/runninscared/2011/01/should_you_get.php.

Douglas, Susan J., and Meredith W. Michaels. *The Mommy Myth: The Idealization of Motherhood and How It Has Undermined Women.* New York: The Free Press, 2004.

Douglas, Susan J., and Meredith W. Michaels. *The Mommy Myth: The Idealization of Motherhood and How It Has Undermined Women.* New York: Free Press, 2004.

Dowling, Amber. "Pregnancy ruins good TV." *TVguideca.* n.d. http://tvguide.ca/home/ (accessed April 2007).

Duden, Barbara. *Disembodying Women: Perspectives on Pregnancy and the Unborn.* Cambridge: Harvard University Press, 1993.

Duhigg, Charles. "How Companies Learn Your Secrets." *New York Times Magazine,* February 16, 2012. http://www.nytimes.com/2012/02/19/magazine/shopping-habits.html?pagewanted=all.

Eastman, Nicholas J. *Expectant Motherhood.* Boston: Little, Brown and Company, 1957.

Eckard, Paul Gallant. *Maternal Body and Voice in Toni Morrison, Bobbie Ann Mason, and Lee Smith.* Columbia, MO: University of Missouri Press, 2002.

Eckard, Paula Gallant. *Maternal Body and Voice in Toni Morrison, Bobbie Ann Mason, and Lee Smith.* Columbia, MO: University of Missouri Press, 2002.

Eckhholm, Erick, and Kim Severson. "Other States Take Notice of Measure on Abortion." *New York Times,* February 29, 2012: Academic Search Premier (Access No. 72085435).

Eggers, Dave, and Vendela Vida. *Away We Go.* Directed by Sam Mendes. Produced by Focus Features. Universal City, CA. 2009.

Eisenberg, Ziv. "Clear and Pregnant Danger: The Making of Prenatal Psychology in Mid-Twentieth Century America." *Journal of Women's History* 22, no. 3 (2010): 112–35.

Ellie & Melissa, The Baby Planners. n.d. Ellie & Melissa, The Baby Planners, http://www.thebabyplanners.com.

Enjoy Your Digital Life. *The Gestation Project.* n.d. http://www.enjoyyourdigitallife.com/the-gestation-project/ (accessed August 29, 2006).

Farrell, Noreen, Jamie Dolkas, and Mia Munro. "Expecting a Baby, Not a Lay-Off: Why Federal Law Should Require The Reasonable Accommodation of Pregnant Workers." *Equal Rights Advocates.* May 10, 2012. http://www.equalrights.org/media/2012/ERA-PregAccomReport.pdf.

Feinstein, Richard J. "Ovary Action." *King of Queens.* Season 4, episode 12, directed by Rob Schiller, aired December 17, 2001 (CBS).

Fey, Tina, and Jack Burditt. "Jack Meets Dennis." *30 Rock.* Season 1, episode 6, directed by Juan José Campanella, aired November 30, 2006 (NBC).

Finestra, Carmen, Gary Kott, and John Markus. "The Day the Spores Landed." *The Cosby Show.* Season 6, Episode 8, directed by Neema Barnette, aired November 9, 1989.

Fisch, Harry. *The Male Biological Clock: The Startling News about Aging, Sexuality, and Fertility in Men.* New York: Free Press, 2005.

Fissell, Mary E. *Vernacular Bodies: The Politics of Reproduction in Early Modern England.* New York: Oxford University Press, 2004.

Fothergill, W. E. *Manual of Midwifery: For the Use of Students and Practitioners.* New York: The Macmillan Company, 1896.

Franklin, Jeff, and Boyd Hale. "Rock the Cradle." *Full House.* Season 4, episode 26, directed by Joel Zwick, aired May 3, 1991 (ABC).

Ganz, Lowell, and Babaloo Mandel. *Parenthood.* Directed by Ron Howard. Produced by Universal. Los Angeles, CA. 1989.

Gélis, Jacques. *History of Childbirth: Fertility, Pregnancy, and Birth in Early Modern Europe.* Translated by Rosemary Morris. Cambridge, UK: Polity Press, 1991.

Genzinger, Neil. "Painful Baby Boom on Primetime TV." *New York Times,* November 2, 2011. http://www.nytimes.com/2011/11/03/arts/television/harrowing-births-on-prime-time-tv.html?pagewanted=all (accessed November 2, 2011).

Ginty, Molly M. "Female Troubles for Wildlife Raise Human Worries." *Women's eNews.* December 18, 2006. http://womensenews.org/story/environment/061218/female-troubles-wildlife-raise-human-worries.

Godshall, Liberty, and Ann Lewis Hamilton. "Love and Sex." *Thirtysomething.* Season 3, episode 2, directed by Marshall Herskovitz, aired October 3, 1989 (ABC).

Goodwin-Kelly, Mary Kate. "Pregnant Body and/As Smoking Gun." In *Motherhood Misconceived,* edited by Heather Addison, Mary Kate Goodwin-Kelly and Elaine Roth, 15–28. Albany: State University of New York Press, 2009.

Gootman, Elissa. "Honey, the Baby is Coming; Quick, Call the Photographer." *New York Times,* June 17, 2012, Late ed.: A1, A14.

Gootman, Elissa. "So Eager for Grandchildren, They're Paying the Egg-Freezing Clinic." *New York Times,* May 13, 2012.

Grant, Julia. *Raising Baby by the book: the Education of American Mothers.* New Haven: Yale University Press, 1998.

Green, Clara Totenberg. "Nebraska Laws Ban Abortions Based on Fetal Pain, Challenging 35 Years of Constitutionally Protected Reproductive Freedom." *Legal Momentum, The Women's Legal Defense and Education Fund.* April 20, 2010. http://legalmomentum.typepad.com/blog/2010/04/nebraska-laws-ban-abortions-based-on-fetal-pain-challenging-35-years-of-constitutionally-protected-r.html.

Greenstein, Jeff, and Jeff Strauss. "The One with the Birth." *Friends.* Season 1, episode 23, directed by James Burrows, aired May 11, 1995 (NBC).

"Gwyneth Paltrow and Bryce Dallas Howard Describe Postpartum Depression." *Huffington Post.* July 22, 2010. http://www.chicagomanualofstyle.org/16/ch14/ch14_sec200.html.

Hackett, Albert, Frances Goodrich, Nancy Meyers, and Charles Shyer. *Father of the Bride Part II.* Directed by Charles Shyer. Produced by Buena Vista. Burbank, CA. 1995.

Hamilton, Ann Lewis. "New Baby." *Thirtysomething.* Season 3, episode 4, directed by Marshall Herskovitz, aired October 24, 1989 (ABC).

Hampton, Brenda. "Falling in Love." *The Secret Life of the American Teenager.* Season 1, episode 1, directed by Ron Underwood, aired September 3, 2008 (ABC Family).

Hampton, Brenda. "It Takes Two, Baby." *7th Heaven.* Season 3, episode 1, directed by Burt Brinckerhoff, aired September 21, 1998 (WB).

Hampton, Brenda, and Jeffrey Rodgers. "Paper or Plastic." *7th Heaven.* Season 9, episode 12, directed by Michael Preece, aired January 24, 2005 (WB).

Hanson, Clare. *A Cultural History of Pregnancy: Pregnancy, Medicine and Culture, 1750–2000.* New York: Palgrave Macmillan, 2004.

Harmon, Amy. "Couples Cull Embryos to Halt Heritage of Cancer." *New York Times,* September 3, 2006.

Harmon, Amy. "Genetic Testing + Abortion=???" *New York Times,* May 13, 2007.

Hearst Corporation. *womansday.com.* n.d. http://www.womansday.com/.

Henricks, Jennifer. "The Magician's Code: Part 1." *How I Met Your Mother.* Season 7, episode 23, directed by Pamela Fryman, aired May 14, 2012 (CBS).

Higginbotham, Abraham, and Dan O'Shannon. "Aunt Mommy." *Modern Family.* Season 3, episode 15, directed by Michael Spiller, aired February 15, 2012 (ABC).

High, Kamau. "Pregnancy Test's Clearblue Odyssey." *Adweek,* December 18, 2006.

Hochschild, Arlie Russell. *The Outsourced Life: Intimate Life in Market Times.* New York: Metropolitan Books, 2012.

Hockschild, Arlie Russell. *The Second Shift.* New York: Penguin Books, 2003.

Hoffert, Sylvia D. *Private matters: American Attitudes toward Childbearing and Infant Nurture in the Urban North, 1800–1860.* Chicago: University of Illinois Press, 1989.

"Homebirth with a Side of Placenta." *Pregnant in Heels.* Season 2, episode 1, aired May 15, 2012 (Bravo).

Howe, Neil, and William Strauss. *Millennials Rising: The Next Great Generation.* New York: Vintage Books, 2000.

Hughes, John. *She's Having a Baby.* Directed by John Hughes. Produced by Paramount Pictures. Hollywood, CA. 1988.

Hulbert, Ann. *Raising America: Experts, Parents, and a Century of Advice About Children.* New York: Alfred A. Knopf, 2003.

Humber, James M., and Robert F. Almeder. *Reproduction, Technology, and Rights.* Totowa, NJ: Humana Press, 1996.

I Didn't Know I was Pregnant. Seasons 1–4, 2008–2011 (TLC).

I'm pregnant and. . . . Seasons 1 and 2, 2009–2011 (Discovery Health).

Iovine, Vicki. *The Girlfriends' Guide to Pregnancy.* New York: Pocket Books, 1999.

"It's A Boy: War Reporter's Baby Shower in Baghdad." *NPR's Morning Edition,* July 6, 2010. http://www.npr.org/templates/story/ story.php?storyId=128061606NPR.org.

"Jennifer." *Sixteen and Pregnant.* Aired July 23 2009 (MTV).

"Jennifer Lopez's Baby Shower." *AskMen.Com Newsletter,* January 18, 2008. http://www.askmen.com/celebs/entertainment-news/jennifer-lopez/jennifer-lopezs-baby-shower.html.

Jordan, Brigitte. *Birth in Four Cultures: A Crosscultural Investigation of Childbirth in Yucatan, Holland, Sweden, and the United States.* Prospect Heights, IL: Waveland Press, Inc., 1993.

Josefsberg, Milt, and Ben Starr. "Gloria is Nervous." *All in the Family.* Season 6, episode 13, directed by Paul Bogart, aired December 8, 1975 (CBS).

Joyce, Amy. "Pregnancy Case Yields Payout of $48.9 million." *Washington Post,* June 6, 2006.

Juzwiak, Rich. "Examining VH1 Dad Camp With Dr. Jeff—Episode 1." *VH1Blog,* May 31, 2010. http://blog.vh1.com/2010–05–31/examining-vh1-dad-camp-with-dr-jeff-episode-1/.

Kao USA (Curel). n.d. http://www.curel.com/pregnancy (accessed January 2010).

Kaplan, E. Ann. *Motherhood and Representation: The Mother in Popular Culture and Melodrama.* New York: Routledge, 1992.

Karger, Dave. "Angelina Jolie: A Candid Q&A." *EW.com Entertainment Weekly.* June 11, 2008. http://www.ew.com/ew/article/0,,20205854,00.html.

Katims, Jason. "Nora." *Parenthood.* Season 3, episode 5 directed by Allison Liddi-Brown, aired October 11, 2011 (NBC).

Kiley, David. "Carl's Jr. Fetus Ads Creepier than a Jr. High School Health Film." *Bloomberg Business Week*. April 11, 2005. http://www.businessweek.com/the_thread/ brandnewday/archives/2005/04/carls_jr_fetus.html.

Kline, Kimberly. "Midwife Attended Births in Prime-Time television: Craziness, Controlling Bitches, and Ultimate Capitulation." *Women & Language* 30, no. 1 (Spring 2007): 20–29.

Kolata, Gina. "Pregnant Exercisers Test Limits." *New York Times*, November 8, 2007: G1, G8.

Kolker, Claudia. *The Immigrant Advantage: What We Can Learn from Newcomers to America about Health, Happiness and Hope.* New York: Free Press, 2011.

Kramer, Steven Philip. "Mind the Baby Gap." *New York Times*, April 18, 2012. http://www.nytimes.com/2012/04/19/opinion/mind-the-baby-gap.html (accessed April 18, 2012).

Kuchinskas, Susan. "All the World's a GoldenPalace.com." *Internetnews.com*. June 1, 2005. http://www.internetnews.com/ec-news/article.php/3508966/All+the+Worlds+a+GoldenPalacecom.htm.

Kuczynski, Alex. "The Nine Months of Living Anxiously." *New York Times*, May 23, 2004: section 9.

Kukla, Rebecca. *Mass Hysteria: Medicine, Culture, and Mothers' Bodies.* New York: Rowman and Littlefield, 2005.

Kushner, Tony, and Eric Roth. *Munich.* Directed by Steven Spielberg. Produced by Universal. Universal City, CA. 2005.

Kutulas, Judy. "'Do I Look Like a Chick'?: Men, women, and Babies on Sitcom Maternity Stories." *American Studies*, Summer 1998: 13–32.

La Ferla, Ruth. "Showing? It's Time to Show Off." *New York Times*, June 8, 2006: G1.

Leavitt, Sarah A. "'A Private Little Revolution': The Home Pregnancy Test in American Culture." *Bulletin of the History of Medicine* 80, no. 2 (Summer 2006): 317–45.

Leavitt, Sarah A. "A Thin Blue Line: A History of the Pregnancy Test Kit." *Stetten Museum, Office of NIH History.* December 2003. http://history.nih.gov/exhibits/thinblueline/index.html.

Leavitt, Sarah A., and Judith Walzer. *Make Room for Daddy: The Journey from Waiting Room to Birthing Room.* Chapel Hill: University of North Carolina Press, 2009.

Leeds, Howard. "A Very Special Delivery." *Bewitched.* Season 2, episode 2, directed by William Asheraired, September 23, 1965 (ABC).

Levin, Ira, and Roman Polanski. *Rosemary's Baby.* Directed by Roman Polanski. Produced by Paramount Pictures. Los Angeles, CA. 1968.

Levine, Ken. "Bravo's Pregnant in Heels—Oh My Fucking God!" *The World as Seen by a TV Comedy Writer, (Blog).* April 6, 2011. http://kenlevine.blogspot.com/2011/04/bravos-pregnant-in-heels-oh-my-fucking.html (accessed May 30, 2012).

Libby, Sara. "Is Forever 21 Glamorizing Teen Pregnancy?" *Salon,* July 20, 2010. http://www.salon.com/2010/07/20/forever_21_maternity/.

Lindhome, Riki, and Kate Micucci. *Pregnant Women are Smug.* Performed by Garfunkel and Oats. http://www.youtube.com/watch?v=tJRzBpFjJS8. n.d.

Lippman, Abby. "The Genetic Construction of Prenatal Testing: Choice, Consent, or Conformity for Women?" In *Women and Prenatal Testing: Facing the Challenges of Genetic Technology,* edited by Karen H. Rothenberg and Elizabeth J. Thomson, 9–34. Columbus, OH: Ohio State University Press, 1994.

Lipsitz, Rebecca. "Pregnancy Tests." *Scientific American* 283, no. 5 (November 2000): 110–12.

Liptak, Adam. "Putting the Government's Words in the Doctor's Mouth." August 6, 2007.

Litke, Cara. "Pregnant Chicks Who Brag Too Much." *Cosmopolitan.* n.d. http://www.cosmopolitan.com/advice/tips/pregnant-chicks-who-brag-too-much (accessed August 21, 2011).

Loeb, Allan, and Jeffrey Eugenides. *The Switch.* Directed by Josh Gordon and Will Speck. Produced by Miramax. Santa Monica, CA. 2010.

Long, Camilla. "Bumponomics." *Sunday Times (London),* May 13, 2012: Style section.

Lynch, David. *Eraserhead.* Directed by David Lynch. Produced by American Film Institute. Los Angeles, CA. 1977.

Mactavish, Scott. *The New Dad's Survival Guide: Man-to-Man Advice for First-Time Fathers.* New York: Little, Brown and Company, 2005.

Marcotte, Amanda. "Randall Terry's Self-Promoting Super Bowl Fetus Ads." *Guardian (Manchester).* January 12, 2012. http://www.guardian.co.uk/commentisfree/cifamerica/2012/jan/12/randall-terry-super-bowl-fetus-ads.

Mario Lopez: Saved by the Baby. Season 1, 2010 (VH1).

Maternity Center Association. *Routines for Maternity Nursing and Briefs for Mothers Club Talks.* New York: Maternity Center Association, 1935.

Matthews, Sandra, and Laura Wexler. *Pregnant Pictures.* New York: Routledge, 2000.

Mazzoni, Cristina. *Maternal Impressions: Pregnancy and Childbirth in Literature and Theory.* Ithaca, NY: Cornell University Press, 2002.

McCarthy, Jenny. *Belly Laughs: The Naked Truth about Pregnancy and Childbirth.* Cambridge, MA: Perseus Books, 2006.

McCullers, Michael. *Baby Mama.* Directed by Michael McCullers. Produced by Universal. Universal City CA. 2008.

McLuhan, Marshall. *Understanding Media: The Extensions of Man.* New York: The New American Library, Inc., 1964.

McMillen, Sally G. *Motherhood in the Old South: Pregnancy, Childbirth, and Infant Rearing.* Baton Rouge, LA: Louisiana State University Press, 1990.

Meredith Corporation. www.parents.com. n.d. http://www.parents.com/.

Mirkinson, Jack. "Megyn Kelly Demolishes Mike Gallagher for Calling Her Maternity Leave a 'Racket'." *Huffington Post.* August 9, 2011. http://www.huffingtonpost.com/2011/08/09/megyn-kelly-mike-gallagher-maternity-leave_n_922393.html.

Moore, Frazier. "50 Years Later, Mary Kay and Johnny Recall TV's First Sitcom." *The Columbia,* November 17, 1997: B7.

Murkoff, Heide, Arlene Eisenberg, and Sandee Hathaway. *What to Expect When You're Expecting.* New York: Workman Publishing, 2002.

Murphy, Gary. "Julie and Eric's Baby." *Notes from the Underbelly.* Season 1, episode 5, directed by Barry Sonnenfeld,, aired May 2, 2007 (ABC).

Navaroo, Mireya. "Here Comes the Mother-to-Be." *New York Times,* March 13, 2005: section 9, 1.

New Hope Fertility Center. "The Biological Clock." *New Hope Fertility Center.* n.d. http://72.47.206.49/biological-clock.shtml (accessed September 10, 2010).

Newman, Andrew Adam. "Maker of Pregnancy Test Finds Opportunity in Personal Stories." *New York Times,* May 2, 2010. http://www.nytimes.com/2010/05/03/business/media/03adco.html.

Notes from the Underbelly. Season 1, 2007 (ABC).

Oakley, Ann. *The Captured Womb: A History of the Medical Care of Pregnant Women.* New York: Basil Blackwell, Inc., 1984.

Oaks, Laury. "Smoke-Filled Wombs and Fragile Fetuses: The Social Politics of Fetal Representation." *Signs: Journal of Women in Culture and Society* 26, no. 1 (2000): 63–108.

O'Bannon, Dan. *Alien.* Directed by Ridley Scott. Produced by 20th Century Fox. Century City, CA. 1979.

O'Dell, Jolie. "Facebook adds Pregnancy Profile option: Let the Ads Begin!" *VentureBeat.* August 1, 2011. http://venturebeat.com/2011/08/01/facebook-pregnant/.

Odent, Michel. *The Farmer and the Obstetrician.* New York: Free Association Books, 2002.

Oppenheimer, Jessica, Madelyn Davis, and Bob Caroll, Jr. "Lucy is Enceinte." *I Love Lucy.* Season 2, episode 10, directed by William Asher, aired December 8, 1952 (CBS).

Orenstein, Catherine. *Little Red Riding Hood Uncloaked: Sex, Morality, and the Evolution of a Fairy Tale.* New York: Basic Books, 2002.

Panaritis, Maria. "Children's Clothier Hartstrings Declares Bankruptcy." *Philadelphia Inquirer,* June 4, 2011: A07.

Paul, Anju Mary. "Pregnant Bellies Auctioned as Ad Space on eBay." *Women's eNews.* March 19, 2006. http://womensenews.org/story/ business/ 060319/pregnant-bellies-auctioned-ad-space-ebay (accessed January 23, 2010).

Paul, Annie Murphy. "The First Ache." *New York Times Magazine,* February 10, 2008: 49.

Paul, Annie Murphy. "Too Fat and Pregnant: the maternal risks of obesity." *New York Times*, July 13, 2008: 19.

Paul, Annie Murphy. *Origins: How the Nine Months Before Birth Shape the Rest Of Our Lives*. New York: Free Press, 2010.

Paul, Pamela. *Parenting Inc.* New York: Henry Holt, 2008.

Peeonastick.com. n.d. http://www.peeonastick.com (accessed June 22, 2012).

People. July 12, 2006.

People Magazine. July 12, 2006.

People Weekly. July 29, 1974: 24.

People Weekly. May 27, 1974: 42.

People Weekly. June 10, 1974.

People Weekly. June 3, 1974: 35.

People Weekly. June 10, 1974: 24,19.

People Weekly. "Mailbag." August 18, 2003: 4.

People Weekly. "Medics." June 10, 1974: 33.

People Weekly. "Medics." June 10, 1974: 33.

People Weekly. "Mother Mill." May 5, 1974: 42.

Plan the Perfect Baby Shower. n.d. http://www.plan-the-perfect-baby-shower.com/celebrity-baby-showers.html.

Poggi, Jeanine. "As 'Jersey Shore' Drifts, MTV promotes pregnant Snooki." *Ad Age*. April 27, 2012. http://adage.com/article/special-report-tv-upfront/jersey-shore-drifts-mtv-promotes-pregnant-snooki/234423/.

Pollack, Andrew. "DNA Blueprint for Fetus Built Using Tests of Parents." *New York Times*, June 6, 2012.

Postman, Neil. *Amusing Ourselves to Death: Public Discourse in the Age of Show Business*. New York: Penguin Books, 1985.

Postman, Neil. *Technopoly: The Surrender of Culture to Technology*. New York: Knopf, 1992.

Potter, Ned. "Parents Make Facebook Page for Unborn Child: Becomes Online Journal." *ABC News*. June 2, 2011. http://abcnews.go.com/Technology/facebook-page-unborn-baby-marriah-greene-texas-page/story?id=13734579#.T-BZRvXNmPM.

Powdthavee, Nattavudh. "Think Having Children Will Make You Happy?" *The Psychologist, Online Journal of the British Psychological Society* 22, part 4, April 2009. http://www.thepsychologist.org.uk/archive/archive_home.cfm?volumeID=22&editionID=174&ArticleID=1493.

Pregnancy-Info.net. n.d. http://www.pregnancy-info.net/.

Pregnant in Heels. Seasons 1 and 2, 2011 and 2012 (Bravo).

Pretty Pushers. n.d. http://www.prettypushers.com/.

Price, Jeffrey, Peter S. Seaman, Chris Miller, and Aron Warner. *Shrek the Third*. Directed by Chris Miller and Aron Warner. Produced by Paramount Pictures. Hollywood, CA. 2007.

Rabin, Roni Caryn. "With New Test, Men Can Have At-Home Fertility Screening." *New York Times,* June 4, 2007: A12.

"Race, Gender, and the American Mother: Political Speech and the Maternity Episodes of I Love Lucy and Murphy Brown." *American Studies* 39, no. 2 (Summer 1998): 33–63.

Reback, Katherine. *Fools Rush In.* Directed by Andy Tennant. Produced by Columbia Pictures. Culver City, CA. 1997.

Reed, Richard K. *Birthing Fathers: The Transformation of Men in American Rites of Birth.* New Brunswich, NJ: Rutgers University Press, 2005.

Reiner, Carl. "Where Did I Come From?" *The Dick Van Dyke Show.* Season 1, episode 19, directed by John Rich, aired January 3, 1962 (CBS).

Rhimes, Shonda, and Stacy McKee. "What Have I Done to Deserve This." *Grey's Anatomy.* Season 2, episode 19, directed by Wendy Stanzler, aired February 26, 2006 (NBC).

Richey, Warren. "Old Maternity Leave Won't Count toward Pensions." *Christian Science Monitor,* May 18, 2009.

Rifkind, Hugo. "Brad Pitt and Angelina Joli in London Yesterday." *Times (London),* January 26, 2006: accessed Newspaper Source, Access no. 7EH1515724538.

Rivers, Joan, and Jay Redack. *Rabbit Test.* Directed by Joan Rivers. Produced by AVCO Embassy Pictures, Culver City, CA. 1978.

Rothenberg, Karen. "The Tentative Pregnancy." In *Women and Prenatal Testing: Facing the Challenges of Genetic Technology,* edited by Karen H. Rothenberg and Elizabeth J. Thomson. Columbus, OH: Ohio State University Press, 1994.

Sack, Kevin. "In Ultrasound, Abortion Fight Has New Front." *New York Times,* May 28, 2010.

Safire, William. "'Bump', On Language." *New York Times Magazine,* May 14, 2006: 22.

Saha, Sukanta, et al. "Advanced Paternal Age Is Associated with Impaired Neurocognitive Outcomes during Infancy and Childhood." *PLoS Med* 6, no. 3 (2009): e1000040. doi:10.1371/journal.pmed.10000.

Santora, Marc. "In Fetal Photos, New Developments." *New York Times,* May 17, 2004.

Schink, Peter, and Charles Scott Stewart. *Legion.* Directed by Scott Charles Stewart. Produced by Screen Gems. Culver City CA. 2009.

Scott Baio is 46 . . . and Pregnant. Season 2, 2008 (VH1).

Searle, Thomas. *A Companion for the Season of Maternal Solicitude.* New York: Moore and Paynel, Clinton Hall, 1834.

Segal, Shira. "Homebirth Advocacy on the Internet." *Rupkatha Journal on Interdisciplinary Studies in Humanities.* 2, no. 1 (2010). http://www.rupkatha.com/homebirthvdvocacy.php.

Sharp, Jane. *The Midwives Book Or the Whole Art of Midwifry Discovered: Directing Childbearing Women How to Behave Themselves.* London, New York: Simon Miller, Reprint, by Garland Publishing, Inc., 1671, 1985.

Shelly, Adrienne. *Waitress.* Directed by Adrienne Shelly. Produced by Fox Searchlight. Century City, CA. 2007.

Shields, Brooke. *Down Came the Rain: My Journey Through Postpartum Depression.* New York: Hyperion Press, 2005.

Father of the Bride Part II. Directed by Charles Shyer. Produced by Buena Vista, Burbank, CA. 1995.

Sixteen and Pregnant. Seasons 1–5, 2009–2012 (MTV).

Slade, Bernard. "And Then There Were Three." *Bewitched.* Season 2, episode 18, directed by William Asher, aired January 13, 1966 (ABC).

Smeal, Sylvia. *Unlike the Elephant.* London: Astra Books, 1951.

Smith, Jeremy Adam. *The Daddy Shift. How Stay-at-Home Dads, Breadwinning Moms, and Shared Parenting are Transforming the American Family.* Boston: Beacon Press, 2009.

Solinger, Rickie. *Pregnancy and Power: A Short History of Reproductive Politics in America.* New York: New York University Press, 2005.

Spar, Deborah L. *The Baby Business. How Money, Science, and Politics Drive the Commerce of Conception.* Boston: Harvard Business School Publishing, 2006.

Springen, Karen. "No Candid Camera." *Newsweek,* February 20, 2006: 16.

Stamford and West Hartford Prenatal Imaging Centers. "Advertisement for Fetal Fotos." n.d.

Star, Darren. "Beach Blanket Brandon." *Beverly Hills 90210.* Season 2, episode 1, directed by Charles Braverman, aired July 11, 1991 (FOX).

Starr, Paul. *The Creation of the Media: Political Origins of Modern Communications.* New York: Basic Books, 2004.

Stonyfield Farm. "Stonyfield Farm Introduces First Yogurt for Expectant, Nursing, and New Moms and Beyond." *PRLog.* January 18, 2008. http://www.prlog.org/10046450-stonyfield-farm-introduces-first-yogurt-for-expectant-nursing-and-new-moms-and-beyond.html.

Tahmincioglue, Eve. "Pregnant Workers Filing More Complaints of Bias." *New York Times,* September 14, 2003: section 10.

Tauber, Michelle. "The Private World of Katie Holmes." *People Magazine,* April 24, 2006: 69.

Taylor, Janelle S. "A Fetish Is Born: Sonographers and the Making of the Public Fetus." In *Consuming Motherhood,* by Janelle S Taylor, edited by Janelle S. Taylor, Linda L. Layne, and Danielle F. Wozniak, 187–210. New Brunswick, NJ: Rutgers University Press, 2004.

Taylor, Janelle S. "Image of Contradiction: Obstetrical Ultrasound in American Culture." In *Reproducing Reproduction: Kinship, Power and Technological Innovation,* edited by Sarah Franklin and Helena Ragone Taylor, 15–33. Philadelphia: University of Pennsylvania Press, 1997.

Taylor, Janelle S. "The Public Fetus and the Family Car: From Abortion Politics to a Volvo Advertisement." *Public Culture* 4, no. 2 (Spring 1992).

Thomson-DeVeaux, Amelia. "Guys' Biological Clocks are Ticking Too?" *Equal Writes,* April 7, 2009. http://equalwrites.org/2009/04/07/guys-biological-clocks-are-ticking-too/.

Thurer, Shari. *The Myths of Motherhood: How Culture Reinvents the Good Mother.* New York: Penguin Books, 1994.

Tia & Tamara. Seasons 1 and 2, 2011 and 2012 (Style Network).

"Too Shaky for the Baby." *Tori & Dean.* Season 1, episode 2, directed by Robert Sizemore, aired May 27, 2007 (Oxygen).

Tropp, Laura. "Faking a Sonogram: Representations of Motherhood on Sex and the City." *Journal of Popular Culture* 39, no. 5 (2006).

Tropp, Laura. "Off Their Rockers: Representation of Postpartum Depression." In *Mental Illness in Popular Media: Essays on the Representation of Disorders,* edited by Lawrence C. Rubin. Jefferson: McFarland, 2012.

tvfanatic.com. n.d. http://www.tvfanatic.com/ (accessed May 1, 2012).

U.S. Food and Drug Administration. *Radiation-Emitting Products.* n.d. http://www.fda.gov/radiation-emittingproducts/default.htm (accessed July 7, 2007).

Umansky, Lauri. *Motherhood Reconceived: Feminism and the Legacies of the Sixties.* New York: New York University Press, 1996.

UNfoundation.org. "Mexico City: First Female Mayor Prohibits Pregnancy Tests." *Women's International Network News,* Winter 2000: 72.

Urban Dictionary. September 2, 2008. http://www.urbandictionary.com/define.php?term=baby%20bump.

Van Blarcom, Carolyn Conan. *Getting Ready to Be a Mother: Information and Advice for the Young Woman who is Looking forward to Motherhood.* New York: The Macmillan Company, 1937.

Van Dijck, José. *In Vivo: The Cultural Mediations of Biomedical Science.* Edited by Phillip Thrutle and Robert Mitchell. Seattle: University of Washington Press, 2005.

"The Very Moving Day." *All in the Family.* Season 6, episode 1, directed by Paul Bogart, aired September 8, 1975 (CBS).

The View. Season 12, episode 195, aired June 11, 2009 (ABC).

Wallis, Claudia. "The Down Dilemma." *Time Magazine,* November 21, 2005: 65.

WebMD, LLC. www.webmd.com. n.d. http://www.webmd.com/.

Website of Make Way For Baby. n.d. http://www.makewayforbaby.com/babies/ (accessed 2011).

Weil, Elizabeth. "A Wrongful Birth." *New York Times Magazine,* March 12, 2006: 50.

Weithorn, Michael J. "Walk, Man." *King of Queens.* Season 4, episode 1, directed by Rob Schiller, aired September 24, 2001 (CBS).

Wertz, Richard W., and Dorothy C. Wertz. *Lying-In: A History of Childbirth in America.* New York: Free Press, 1977.

Westfeldt, Jennifer. *Friends with Kids.* Directed by Jennifer Westfeldt. Produced by Roadside Attractions. Los Angeles, CA. 2011.

"What About This Offer?" *Starwood Hotels & Resorts Worldwide.* n.d. http://www.starwoodpromos.com/ whotelsbabyme/ (accessed June 25, 2012).

Williams, Alex, and Kate Murphy. "A Boy or Girl? Cut the Cake." *New York Times,* April 8, 2012: 1–2.

Williams, Caroline. "Birth." *Up All Night.* Season 1, episode 6, directed by Randall Einhorn, aired October 19, 2011 (NBC).

Williams, Wheeler, Dorrie. *The Unplanned Pregnancy Book For Teens and College Students.* Virginia Beach, VA: Sparkledoll Productions Publishing, 2004.

"World Exclusive: Matthew & Camila's Baby Boy." *OK Magazine.* July 23, 2008. http://www.okmagazine.com/babies/world-exclusive-matthew-camilas-baby-boy.

Yahoo Inc. *yahoo.com.* n.d. http://www.yahoo.com/.

Zand, Sarvenaz. "Parents Sue over Pregnancy Test Said to Tell Baby's Sex." *ABC News.* February 28, 2006. http://abcnews.go.com/Health/story?id=1668125&page=1#.T-Ea6_XNmPM.

Zapperi, Roberto. *The Pregnant Man.* New York; Chur, Switzerland: Harwood Academic Publishers, 1991.

Zeitchik, Steven. "B&N Nurtures Pregnancy Book." *Publishers Weekly* 251, no. 50 (December 2004).

Index

About the Author

Laura Tropp is an associate professor and chair of the Communication Arts Department at Marymount Manhattan College. She teaches and writes about media history, popular culture, and motherhood. Not surprisingly, her research into pregnancy coincided with the births of her three children, with whom she resides, along with her husband, in New York City.